Contemporary Surgical Clerkships

Series Editor

Adam E. M. Eltorai, Marlborough, USA

This series of specialty-specific books will serve as high-yield, quick-reference reviews specifically for the numerous third- and fourth-year medical students rotating on surgical clerkships. Edited by experts in the field, each book includes concise review content from a senior resident or fellow and an established academic physician. Students can read the text from cover to cover to gain a general foundation of knowledge that can be built upon when they begin their rotation, or they can use specific chapters to review a subspecialty before starting a new rotation or seeing a patient with a subspecialty attending.

These books will be the ideal, on-the-spot references for medical students and practitioners seeking fast facts on diagnosis and management. Their bullet-pointed format, including user-friendly figures, tables and algorithms, make them the perfect quick-reference. Their content breadth covers the most commonly encountered problems in practice, focusing on the fundamental principles of diagnosis and management. Carry them in your white coat for convenient access to the answers you need, when you need them.

Faina Nakhlis
Editor

Breast Surgery Clerkship

A Guide for Senior Medical Students

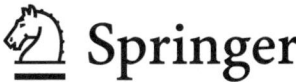

Editor
Faina Nakhlis
Harvard Medical School
Boston, MA, USA

Brigham and Women's Hospital, Division of Breast Surgery
Boston, MA, USA

Dana-Farber Cancer Institute, Breast Oncology Program
Boston, MA, USA

Editorial Contact: Jessica Chio

ISSN 2730-941X   ISSN 2730-9428 (electronic)
Contemporary Surgical Clerkships
ISBN 978-3-032-03949-1   ISBN 978-3-032-03950-7 (eBook)
https://doi.org/10.1007/978-3-032-03950-7

© The Editor(s) (if applicable) and The Author(s), under exclusive license to Springer Nature Switzerland AG 2025

This work is subject to copyright. All rights are solely and exclusively licensed by the Publisher, whether the whole or part of the material is concerned, specifically the rights of translation, reprinting, reuse of illustrations, recitation, broadcasting, reproduction on microfilms or in any other physical way, and transmission or information storage and retrieval, electronic adaptation, computer software, or by similar or dissimilar methodology now known or hereafter developed.
The use of general descriptive names, registered names, trademarks, service marks, etc. in this publication does not imply, even in the absence of a specific statement, that such names are exempt from the relevant protective laws and regulations and therefore free for general use.
The publisher, the authors and the editors are safe to assume that the advice and information in this book are believed to be true and accurate at the date of publication. Neither the publisher nor the authors or the editors give a warranty, expressed or implied, with respect to the material contained herein or for any errors or omissions that may have been made. The publisher remains neutral with regard to jurisdictional claims in published maps and institutional affiliations.

This Springer imprint is published by the registered company Springer Nature Switzerland AG
The registered company address is: Gewerbestrasse 11, 6330 Cham, Switzerland

If disposing of this product, please recycle the paper.

Contents

1 Common Benign Breast Lesions 1
   Brigid K. Killelea

2 Atypical Ductal Hyperplasia (ADH), Atypical Lobular
   Hyperplasia (ALH), Lobular Carcinoma In Situ (LCIS),
   Atypical Papilloma 7
   Faina Nakhlis

3 Screening and Diagnostic Imaging 17
   Leah H. Portnow, Sneha S. Shukla, and Zuby Syed

4 Surgical Treatment of Breast Cancer 41
   Claire Morton and Christina Minami

5 Breast Cancer-Related Lymphedema 55
   Erin M. Taylor

Index 63

Chapter 1
Common Benign Breast Lesions

Brigid K. Killelea

Benign Breast Cysts

Simple Cysts

Breast cysts are not uncommon. These lesions are benign, and usually present as smooth, mobile, fluid-filled masses that can be tender to palpation and bothersome or worrisome to patients. Smaller cysts may not be palpable, and only be visible on ultrasound (see Chap. 3). Simple cysts contain fluid, and appear as dark, round, anechoic masses with posterior enhancement on ultrasound. Larger cysts may appear oval in shape on ultrasound, if they are slightly compressed under the weight of the ultrasound probe during scanning. These simple cysts may fluctuate in size each month under hormonal influence. Simple cysts of the breast do not cause cancer or turn into cancer, and patients can be reassured that they are common and not worrisome. In fact, approximately 7% of women present with a palpable cyst at some point in their life [1].

- Asymptomatic, simple cysts do not require treatment or follow-up.
- Larger, symptomatic cysts may be aspirated with ultrasound or palpation guidance; however, patients should be advised that they may recur.
- Fluid that is aspirated from simple cysts is usually straw-colored and should be discarded.
- Aspirate that is blood-tinged is typically sent for cytologic analysis.

B. K. Killelea (✉)
Brigham and Women's Cancer Center, Boston, MA, USA
e-mail: bkillelea@bwh.harvard.edu

© The Author(s), under exclusive license to Springer Nature
Switzerland AG 2025
F. Nakhlis (ed.), *Breast Surgery Clerkship*, Contemporary Surgical Clerkships,
https://doi.org/10.1007/978-3-032-03950-7_1

Complicated Cysts

Complicated cysts appear as fluid-filled masses that are lobulated or have internal septations seen on ultrasound. The wall of a complicated cyst is often thicker than the wall of a simple cyst. Complicated cysts may contain other material that is visible on ultrasound, including calcium deposits or cellular debris. This material may cause internal echoes on ultrasound. The fluid inside complicated cysts can be turbid or cloudy. Complicated cysts may be palpable or may be picked up incidentally on breast ultrasound.

- Complicated cysts are typically assessed either with ultrasound follow-up if small and benign appearing, or with needle aspiration or core biopsy if they appear suspicious.
- If biopsy is benign, no further treatment is indicated provided that the findings are concordant with imaging. Sometimes, 6-month follow-up ultrasound is recommended to document stability.
- Rarely, complicated cysts that appear suspicious or demonstrate cells suggestive of a high-risk lesion on cytology may need to be surgically excised. Excision is usually performed in the OR with wire, seed, etc., localization.

Fibroepithelial Neoplasms

Fibroadenomas

Fibroadenomas are benign masses that contain both epithelial and stromal elements. As opposed to cysts, which contain mostly fluid, fibroadenomas are solid masses.

Histologically, it can be difficult to distinguish between fibroadenoma and phyllodes tumor (see below) on core biopsy; if there is uncertainty, surgical excision is recommended.

- Ultrasound of benign fibroadenomas reveals a solid mass with smooth, regular borders.
- Fibroadenomas are usually seen in younger women and/or during pregnancy. They may grow in response to hormonal fluctuations.
- Fibroadenomas account for the majority of palpable masses in women aged 20 and under [1].

Fibroadenomas typically present as solid, smooth, mobile masses of the breast. Usually, they are stable in size although some of these lesions get smaller over time.

- Small fibroadenomas can be followed clinically with serial ultrasound and clinical examination over a period of time (typically 18–24 months) to document stability, especially if they are not painful.

- Suspected fibroadenomas over 3 cm in size are typically recommended for core biopsy.
- Suspected fibroadenomas that are smaller can be considered for core biopsy if the diagnosis is uncertain on imaging. It is also appropriate to consider a core biopsy for a suspected fibroadenoma of any size.

Approximately 20–25% will continue to grow, causing pain or deformity in the breast.

- Fibroadenomas that are increasing in size and/or bothersome or uncomfortable to the patient should be excised and sent for pathologic review.

Phyllodes Tumors

Phyllodes tumors are uncommon, and account for less than 1% of all breast tumors [2]. Phyllodes tumors are classified as *benign*, *borderline*, or *malignant*, based on pathology. Clinically and pathologically, however, it can be challenging to differentiate fibroadenomas from phyllodes tumors on the basis of the core biopsy. On pathology, stromal features including hypercellularity, atypia, mitotic activity, and the borders of the tumor are considered when making the diagnosis. Prognosis is related to features seen on histology [3]. Phyllodes tumors with poor features for all of these criteria have a worse prognosis. However, even borderline and malignant tumors with some favorable features have a very good prognosis with complete excision [3].

Clinically, phyllodes tumors tend to be larger than fibroadenomas and occur more commonly in older women, with the fifth decade of life being the most prevalent. Malignant phyllodes tumors rarely metastasize to lymph nodes, so axillary staging is not indicated.

Benign Phyllodes

- Histologically well-developed, leaf-like fronds are characteristic of phyllodes tumors.
- Benign phyllodes display increased stromal cellularity.
- Treatment of benign phyllodes is surgical excision with negative margins.
- While the definition of "negative" margins for phyllodes tumors remains controversial, recent data suggest that no pathology ink seen on tumor cells, as is the case for invasive carcinoma, is sufficient with respect to the risk of a subsequent local recurrence.

Borderline Phyllodes

- Treatment of borderline phyllodes is surgical excision with negative margins.

- After surgical excision, borderline and malignant phyllodes tumors recur with equal frequency. The lifetime risk of local recurrence for borderline and malignant phyllodes tumors is approximately 20%.
- The margin considerations for borderline phyllodes tumors are similar to those for their benign counterparts (above).

Malignant Phyllodes

- Distant metastases occur in 10–20% of patients with malignant phyllodes, with a slight propensity for lung metastasis; therefore, a consultation with a breast medical oncologist to ensure appropriate surveillance is warranted.
- Treatment is surgical excision with negative margins.
- There are limited data to support the addition of radiation to reduce the risk of local recurrence; therefore, a consultation with a radiation oncologist is warranted to enable personalized counseling.

Periareolar Abscess

Infected Montgomery's Gland

The ducts of the breast converge behind the nipple and pass through the nipple skin. The pigmented skin around the nipple is the areola. There are sebaceous glands around the ends of breast ducts, superficially under the areolar skin that lubricate the skin during breast feeding. These glands, known as *Montgomery's glands*/tubercles, can be seen and palpated under the skin of the areola.

- When these glands become blocked, infection may develop.
- If caught early, these infections can be treated with oral antibiotics and warm compresses.
- Larger infections require incision and drainage.

Periductal Fistula

Periductal fistula is an infection that communicates between the edge of the areola and the nipple. These lesions are much more common in smokers. Although the etiology is not completely understood, periductal fistula is much more common in smokers. Clinically, patients often present with long history of a cyclic, chronic infection that spontaneously drains, heals, and then becomes reinfected.

- Treatment for periductal fistula is to treat with a course of antibiotics to decrease the size of the active infection, followed by excision of the entire fistula tract with a radially oriented incision, up to and including the tip of the affected nipple [4].
- Incomplete excision usually results in recurrence of the infection.

Nipple Discharge

Nipple discharge is a common breast symptom that affects up to 80% of women [5, 6]. Certain medical conditions and comorbidities have been associated with nipple discharge, including pituitary tumors, hypothalamic lesions, breast and/or skin infections, shingles, hyperprolactinemia, hypothyroidism, trauma to the breast, and kidney disease. Medications, including both prescription and non-prescription and herbal supplements have been associated with nipple discharge, particularly those that inhibit dopamine secretion, elevate prolactin, and/or affect circulating sex hormones.

Benign or physiologic nipple discharge is typically due to benign causes.

- Benign causes include side effects from medications, duct ectasia, pregnancy, and repeated stimulation or manipulation of the breasts or nipples.
- Benign discharge can be clear yellow, white, gray, brown, or green in color.
- Benign nipple discharge usually resolves once the cause is identified and addressed.

Pathologic nipple discharge is seen in response to a pathologic process or lesion in the breast.

- Common causes include papillomas, mastitis, or a breast abscess.
- Less common causes include malignancy, such as ductal carcinoma in situ (DCIS) or invasive breast cancer.
- *Pathologic nipple discharge* is usually *bloody or clear*, *spontaneous*, emanating from a *single duct*, *persistent* and *reproducible* on clinical exam.

Nipple discharge can be either *non-spontaneous*, meaning that it is only evident with manipulation or squeezing of the nipple, or *spontaneous*, which extrudes through the nipple on its own.

- In most cases, non-spontaneous, bilateral nipple discharge is not worrisome.
- Non-spontaneous nipple discharge can increase in quantity with frequent stimulation or nipple squeezing.
- Discharge that can only be elicited with squeezing or manipulation of the nipple is termed "non-spontaneous nipple discharge" and is not clinically concerning.
- Patients with pathologic nipple discharge should undergo a bilateral diagnostic mammogram and a diagnostic ultrasound of the ipsilateral breast to ensure the absence of concomitant breast pathology. If none is found, patients with pathologic nipple discharge should undergo a duct excision.

References

1. Michael Dixon J, editor. ABC of breast diseases. 4th ed. West Sussex: Wiley-Blackwell BMJ Books; 2012.
2. Genco IS, Purohit V, Hackman K, et al. Benign and borderline phyllodes tumors of the breast: clinicopathologic analysis of 205 cases with emphasis on the surgical margin status and local recurrence rate. Ann Diagn Pathol. 2021;51:151708.
3. Spanheimer PM, et al. Long-term outcomes after surgical treatment of malignant/borderline phyllodes tumors of the breast. Ann Surg Oncol. 2019;26:2136–43.
4. Lanin DR. Twenty-two year experience with recurring subareolar abscess and lactiferous duct fistula treated by a single breast surgeon. Am J Surg. 2004;188(4):407–10.
5. Goodson WH, King EB. The breast: comprehensive management of benign and malignant disorders. 3rd ed. St. Louis: W B Saunders; 2004.
6. Santen RJ. Benign breast disease in women. In: Feingold KR, Anawalt B, Blackman MR, Boyce A, Chrousos G, Corpas E, de Herder WW, Dhatariya K, Dungan K, Hofland J, Kalra S, Kaltsas G, Kapoor N, Koch C, Kopp P, Korbonits M, Kovacs CS, Kuohung W, Laferrère B, Levy M, McGee EA, McLachlan R, New M, Purnell J, Sahay R, Shah AS, Singer F, Sperling MA, Stratakis CA, Trence DL, Wilson DP, editors. Endotext [Internet]. MDText.com, Inc.; South Dartmouth: 2018.

Chapter 2
Atypical Ductal Hyperplasia (ADH), Atypical Lobular Hyperplasia (ALH), Lobular Carcinoma In Situ (LCIS), Atypical Papilloma

Faina Nakhlis

Many benign proliferative breast lesions have been described in pathology and surgical literature. Several observational studies have examined the natural history of these lesions, and obtaining higher-quality data on this topic is unlikely. Nevertheless, there are proliferative breast lesions for which the current literature is unanimous regarding the increased future breast cancer risk associated with them. These lesions include atypical ductal hyperplasia, atypical lobular hyperplasia, classic lobular carcinoma in situ, florid lobular carcinoma in situ, pleomorphic lobular carcinoma in situ, and atypical papilloma. Understanding the implications of diagnosing these lesions through core biopsy or excision is crucial to ensure appropriate referral of these patients for breast cancer risk assessment and risk reduction counseling.

Atypical Ductal Hyperplasia (ADH) [1]

Incidence and Epidemiology

Atypical ductal hyperplasia (ADH) is a proliferative breast lesion whose incidence has increased over the last few decades with the growing utilization of screening mammography. It is seen in approximately 14% of image-guided core biopsies. A normal lactiferous duct consists of a single layer of cuboidal epithelium, while ADH

F. Nakhlis (✉)
Harvard Medical School, Boston, MA, USA

Brigham and Women's Hospital, Division of Breast Surgery, Boston, MA, USA

Dana-Farber Cancer Institute, Breast Oncology Program, Boston, MA, USA
e-mail: fnakhlis1@bwh.harvard.edu

is characterized by multiple cell layers exhibiting various degrees of atypia (Fig. 2.1). The extent of atypia may make ADH difficult to distinguish from low-grade ductal carcinoma in situ (DCIS) (Fig. 2.2). The distinction between ADH and low-grade DCIS is based on the following criteria (Table 2.1):

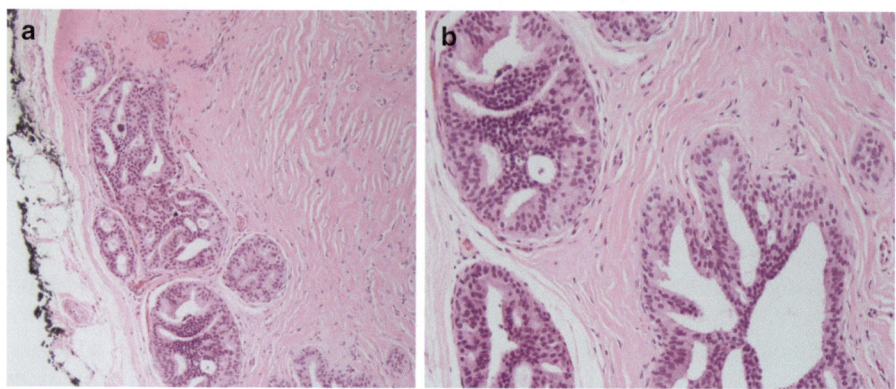

Fig. 2.1 Atypical ductal hyperplasia. Atypical ductal hyperplasia at 10× (**a**) and 20× (**b**). (Courtesy of Dr. Venable, Department of Pathology, Brigham and Women's Hospital, Boston, MA)

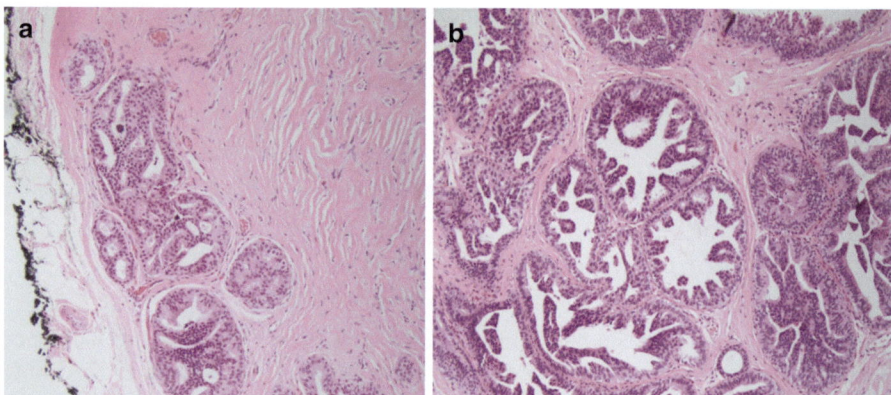

Fig. 2.2 Atypical ductal hyperplasia and low-grade DCIS. Atypical ductal hyperplasia (**a**) and low-grade DCIS (**b**) at 10×. DCIS: ductal carcinoma in situ. (Courtesy of Dr. Venable, Department of Pathology, Brigham and Women's Hospital, Boston, MA)

Table 2.1 Histologic features of atypical ductal hyperplasia (ADH) and ductal carcinoma in situ (DCIS)

	ADH	DCIS
Number of involved ducts	<2	≥2
Size of lesion	<2 mm	≥2 mm

ADH atypical ductal hyperplasia, *DCIS* ductal carcinoma in situ

Core Biopsy Diagnosis of ADH

Due to the histologic resemblance of ADH and DCIS, historically ADH seen on core biopsy was recommended for a larger (excisional or surgical) biopsy to be able to evaluate a sufficiently sizeable tissue sample to rule out DCIS or invasive carcinoma. Earlier technology, which utilized smaller gauge biopsy needles, provided rather little tissue for histologic evaluation, and the likelihood of finding carcinoma on excision of ADH found on core biopsy (also referred to as an "upgrade in diagnosis") was between 25% and 40%. In the latter years, 8–10-gauge biopsy needles have been used to obtain core biopsies, and the likelihood of upgrade has decreased to 10–25%. Nonetheless, the upgrade rate to carcinoma on excision of ADH found on core biopsy is sufficiently high that the standard of care in the management of the latter remains an excisional biopsy.

ADH and Future Breast Cancer Risk Implications

ADH is considered a non-obligate breast cancer precursor based on the existing data. While several observational studies have shown a higher likelihood of developing future breast cancer in the breast ipsilateral to the prior ADH, a definitive breast carcinogenesis model with ADH as an intermediate step does not exist. Furthermore, ipsilateral breast carcinomas can be found anywhere in the affected breast, not necessarily at the prior site of ADH.

- There is a consensus from large observational studies and single-institution series demonstrating an overall elevated future breast cancer risk associated with the diagnosis of ADH. The increase in the lifetime breast cancer risk associated with ADH, compared to that of the general population, is about fourfold, amounting to an estimated breast cancer lifetime risk of 15–20%.
- Considering the elevated lifetime breast cancer risk in patients diagnosed with ADH, these women should undergo appropriate risk counseling and be educated about their breast cancer risk-reducing options. Several agents have been shown to reduce subsequent breast cancer risk in this patient population (Table 2.2).

Table 2.2 Commonly used chemotherapeutic agents for breast cancer risk reduction [2]

Agent	Eligible population	Breast cancer risk reduction magnitude (%)	Side effects
Tamoxifen 20 mg/day × 5 years	Age 35 and older, ADH, ALH, LCIS	31	Hot flashes, endometrial cancer[a], thromboembolic events[a]
Raloxifene 60 mg/day × 5 years	Postmenopausal, ADH, ALH, LCIS	56	Hot flashes
Anastrozole 1 mg/day × 5 years	Postmenopausal, ADH, ALH, LCIS	45	Hot flashes, osteopenia, arthralgias
Exemestane 25 mg/day × 5 years	Postmenopausal, ADH, ALH, LCIS	45	Hot flashes, osteopenia, arthralgias

ADH atypical ductal hyperplasia, *ALH* atypical lobular hyperplasia, *LCIS* lobular carcinoma in situ
[a]In therapeutic and prevention trials of tamoxifen, the risk of endometrial carcinoma and thromboembolic events has been reported to be 0.8% for each, which is approximately four times higher than that of the non-tamoxifen study arms, but overall, it remains relatively low. However, tamoxifen has been avoided in patients with additional risk factors for endometrial carcinoma or thromboembolism. Recently, low-dose tamoxifen (5 mg daily) has shown similar efficacy to the 20 mg daily regimen. To date, the incidence of thromboembolic events and endometrial cancer associated with low-dose tamoxifen administration has been comparable to that of the general population

Lobular Neoplasia (Atypical Lobular Hyperplasia and Classic LCIS) [3, 4]

Incidence and Epidemiology

Lobular neoplasia (LN) is atypical epithelial cell proliferation in the terminal duct lobular unit (TDLU), which includes both atypical lobular hyperplasia (ALH) and classic lobular carcinoma in situ (C-LCIS). Monomorphic dyshesive cells comprise LN, and the distinction between ALH and C-LCIS is quantitative: ALH occupies less than 50% of the TDLU, while C-LCIS is seen in 50% or greater of the TDLU (Fig. 2.3).

- The distinction between C-LCIS and low-grade ductal carcinoma in situ (DCIS) can be challenging. Immunohistochemical staining for E-cadherin in DCIS is typically positive, and ALH, C-LCIS as well as most proliferative lobular lesions are E-cadherin-negative.
- LN is seen in 0.5–3.6% of all core biopsies, does not have clinical presenting symptoms (such as palpable mass or nipple discharge), and most commonly presents as mammographic calcifications although is considered an incidental finding.

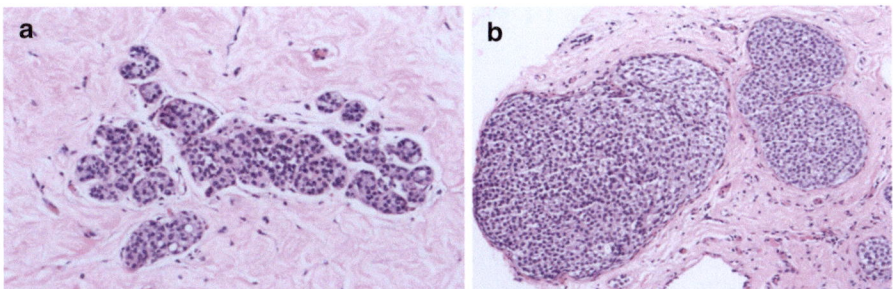

Fig. 2.3 Atypical lobular hyperplasia and classic lobular carcinoma in situ. Atypical lobular hyperplasia (**a**) and classic lobular carcinoma in situ (**b**) at 10×. (Courtesy of Dr. Mashayekhi, Department of Pathology, Brigham and Women's Hospital, Boston, MA)

Core Biopsy Diagnosis of LN [3]

For LN diagnosed on core biopsy of clinically asymptomatic screening breast imaging-detected lesions, the likelihood of finding an adjacent concomitant carcinoma on excisional biopsy is rather low in the recent studies, ranging between 1% and 3%. These data apply to lesions that are classified as Breast Imaging Reporting & Data System (BI-RADS) (see Chap. 3) category 4 or lower and are deemed radiographically pathologically concordant. Considering this, clinical management of core biopsies with LN requires a multidisciplinary approach involving Breast Imaging and Pathology to ensure whether non-surgical management is appropriate.

LN and Future Breast Cancer Risk Implications

ALH and C-LCIS are well known to be associated with an elevated future breast cancer risk.

- Several epidemiologic and population-based studies have shown that the future breast cancer risk is elevated by four- to fivefold in patients with ALH and by eight- to tenfold in those with C-LCIS. Patients diagnosed with LN must be referred for appropriate breast cancer risk education and counseling regarding their breast cancer risk-reducing options (Table 2.2).
- Patients with C-LCIS may benefit the most from chemoprevention. King et al. [4] reported on over 1000 women with C-LCIS prospectively followed at a single institution between 1980 and 2009, with a median follow-up of 82 months years. In this cohort, the only factor associated with breast cancer risk reduction was the receipt of chemoprevention (HR = 0.269, 95% CI 0.15–0.50, $P < 0.001$).

Florid and Pleomorphic LCIS [5]

Incidence and Epidemiology

Florid and pleomorphic LCIS (Fig. 2.4) are rare variants of LCIS that are associated with controversy regarding their definition and natural history. In the past, a multitude of terms was used to refer to these histologic entities, such as variant LCIS, non-classic LCIS, carcinoma in situ with ductal and lobular features, as well as pleomorphic LCIS, florid LCIS, and LCIS with necrosis. This was further complicated by notable interobserver variability when diagnosing these lesions, which has led to many challenges in studying them and formulating reliable management guidance.

Core Biopsy Diagnosis of Florid and Pleomorphic LCIS

As stated above, due to the existing controversy in diagnosing florid and pleomorphic LCIS and the inconsistency of prior terminology utilized to refer to these histologic entities, the data on the upgrade rates to carcinoma found on their excision are rather limited. All the existing literature is retrospective; it includes small numbers collected over many years. Nonetheless, the reported upgrade rates have been quite consistently ranging between 25% and 60%. Based on this, routine excision following a core biopsy diagnosis of florid and pleomorphic LCIS is warranted to rule out an associated carcinoma.

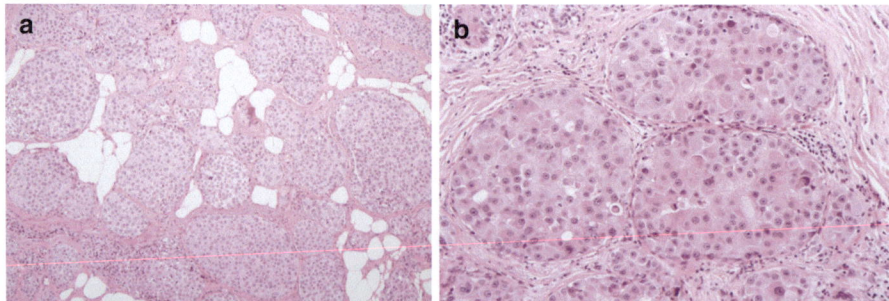

Fig. 2.4 Florid and pleomorphic LCIS. Florid LCIS (**a**) and pleomorphic LCIS (**b**) at 10×. LCIS: lobular carcinoma in situ. (Courtesy of Dr. Mashayekhi, Department of Pathology, Brigham and Women's Hospital, Boston, MA)

Florid and Pleomorphic LCIS and Future Breast Cancer Risk Implications

The data regarding the natural history of florid and pleomorphic LCIS are very scarce, and their interpretation is challenging due to significant variability in the clinical management of the patients with these lesions. Nonetheless, since the majority of florid and pleomorphic LCIS lesions are estrogen-receptor-positive, chemoprevention should be considered in this patient population.

Atypical Papilloma [6]

Incidence and Epidemiology

Papillary breast lesions are encountered in 5–10% of breast biopsies. Their presentation varies from asymptomatic breast imaging-detected masses to palpable masses to pathologic nipple discharge (the latter defined as bloody or clear spontaneous single-duct nipple discharge). Atypical papillomas (Fig. 2.5) contain some degree of concomitant atypical hyperplasia, which can be challenging for pathologists to differentiate from ductal carcinoma in situ. In one of the larger longitudinal series of patients with atypical papillomas, the mean patient age range was 59–65 years.

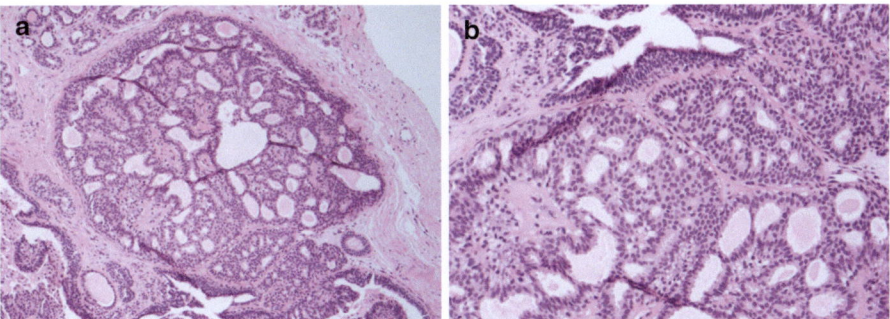

Fig. 2.5 Atypical papilloma. Atypical papilloma at 10× (**a**) and 20× (**b**). (Courtesy of Dr. Venable, Department of Pathology, Brigham and Women's Hospital, Boston, MA)

Core Biopsy Diagnosis of Atypical Papilloma

A meta-analysis by Wen and Cheng evaluated 34 studies, which included over 2000 breast papillomas on core biopsy, of which over 600 were atypical. Among the latter group, the upgrade rate to carcinoma on excision was 37%. In contrast to that, the upgrade rate on excision of BI-RADS≤4 asymptomatic papillomas without atypia, the upgrade rate on excision is 1.7%.

Atypical Papilloma and Future Breast Cancer Risk Implications

Lewis et al. [7] reported the natural history of various proliferative breast lesions in patients longitudinally followed at the Mayo Clinic. Among them, there were 54 patients with a solitary atypical papilloma, and 13 patients with multiple atypical papillomas. In the former group, 12 patients developed breast cancer over 6.2 years of mean follow-up, while in the latter 4 breast cancer diagnoses were documented over 5.8 years of mean follow-up. Based on these observations, the relative risk of breast cancer development associated with solitary atypical papillomas was 5.11 (95% CI 2.64–8.92), while that with multiple atypical papillomas was 7.01 (95% CI 1.91–17.97).

On the basis of these risk estimates, these patients should be appropriately counseled, and chemoprevention should be discussed.

References

1. Zaveri S, Sun SX, Zaghloul T, Bevers TB, et al. Trends in atypical ductal hyperplasia diagnosis and upgrade: a 20-year experience and impact of MRI use on upgrade rates. Ann Surg Oncol. 2025;32:3244–51. https://doi.org/10.1245/s10434-025-16933-6. Epub ahead of print. PMID: 39875718.
2. Nelson HD, Fu R, Zakher B, Pappas M, McDonagh M. Medication use for the risk reduction of primary breast cancer in women: updated evidence report and systematic review for the US Preventive Services Task Force. JAMA. 2019;322(9):868–86. https://doi.org/10.1001/jama.2019.5780. PMID: 31479143.
3. Nakhlis F, Gilmore L, Gelman R, Bedrosian I, et al. Incidence of adjacent synchronous invasive carcinoma and/or ductal carcinoma in-situ in patients with lobular neoplasia on core biopsy: results from a prospective multi-institutional registry (TBCRC 020). Ann Surg Oncol. 2016;23(3):722–8. https://doi.org/10.1245/s10434-015-4922-4. Epub 2015 Nov 5. PMID: 26542585; PMCID: PMC4984674.
4. King TA, Pilewskie M, Muhsen S, Patil S, et al. Lobular carcinoma in situ: a 29-year longitudinal experience evaluating clinicopathologic features and breast cancer risk. J Clin Oncol. 2015;33(33):3945–52. https://doi.org/10.1200/JCO.2015.61.4743. Epub 2015 Sept 14. PMID: 26371145; PMCID: PMC4934644.

5. Schnitt SJ, Brogi E, Chen YY, King TA, Lakhani SR. American registry of pathology expert opinions: the spectrum of lobular carcinoma in situ: diagnostic features and clinical implications. Ann Diagn Pathol. 2020;45:151481. https://doi.org/10.1016/j.anndiagpath.2020.151481. Epub 2020 Feb 15. PMID: 32120324; PMCID: PMC7401835.
6. Wen X, Cheng W. Nonmalignant breast papillary lesions at core-needle biopsy: a meta-analysis of underestimation and influencing factors. Ann Surg Oncol, 2013;20(1):94–101. https://doi.org/10.1245/s10434-012-2590-1. Epub 2012 Aug 10. PMID: 22878621.
7. Lewis JT, Hartmann LC, Vierkant RA, et al. An analysis of breast cancer risk in women with single, multiple, and atypical papilloma. Am J Surg Pathol. 2006;30:665–72.

Chapter 3
Screening and Diagnostic Imaging

Leah H. Portnow, Sneha S. Shukla, and Zuby Syed

Screening in Breast Imaging

Screening Mammography

Breast screening mammography is a critical tool used for the early detection of breast cancer in asymptomatic women, which often leads to earlier intervention, improved prognosis, and reduced mortality [1, 2]. Mammography involves taking X-ray images of the breast to identify abnormalities including calcifications and soft tissue changes of masses, asymmetries, architectural distortion that may indicate the presence of breast cancer. Screening mammography is performed as a standard 4-view examination, with two views of each breast in the craniocaudal (CC) and mediolateral oblique (MLO) projection (Fig. 3.1).

Imaging Views

Breast mammography involves capturing images of the breast from multiple standardized views to ensure thorough evaluation of the tissue. Here is a detailed description of the different views used in mammography:

L. H. Portnow (✉) · S. S. Shukla · Z. Syed
Department of Radiology, Brigham and Women's Hospital, Boston, MA, USA
e-mail: lportnow@bwh.harvard.edu

© The Author(s), under exclusive license to Springer Nature
Switzerland AG 2025
F. Nakhlis (ed.), *Breast Surgery Clerkship*, Contemporary Surgical Clerkships,
https://doi.org/10.1007/978-3-032-03950-7_3

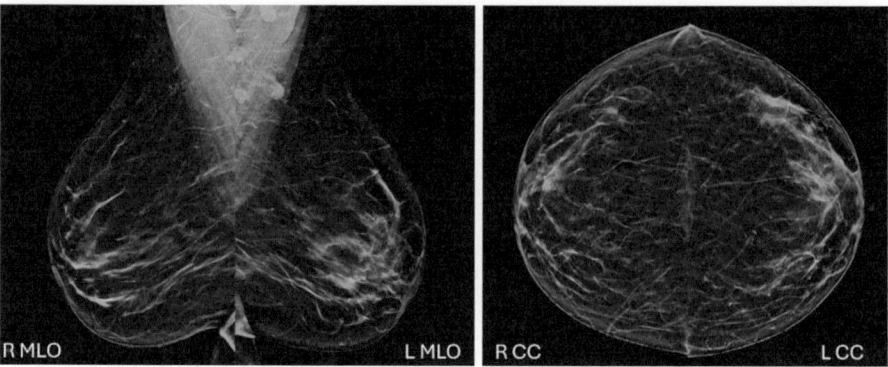

Fig. 3.1 Standard screening mammogram demonstrating mediolateral oblique (MLO) and craniocaudal (CC) views of the right (R) and left (L) breasts. This woman's breast composition is category B: scattered areas of fibroglandular density

Standard Views

View	Description	Purpose	Technique
Craniocaudal (CC)	A top-to-bottom image of the breast	Evaluates the central, inner, and outer breast tissue	The breast is compressed horizontally between two plates. The X-ray beam travels from above (cranial) to below (caudal)
Mediolateral oblique (MLO)	An angled view that includes the upper outer quadrant of the breast and the axillary tail	Provides a comprehensive view of deeper tissues and lymph nodes	The breast is compressed at an angle (40–60°) between the plates. The X-ray beam travels from the inner (medial) side to the outer (lateral) side

Special Views

View	Description	Purpose	Technique
Implant displaced (ID) or Eklund technique	Designed to visualize natural breast tissue in patients with implants	Pushes the implant back while pulling the breast tissue forward	Standard CC and MLO views are taken with and without the implant displaced

Digital Breast Tomosynthesis

Digital breast tomosynthesis (DBT), also known as 3D mammography, is an advanced imaging technique that provides a more detailed, three-dimensional view of the breast compared to traditional 2D mammography. By capturing multiple X-ray images from different angles while the breast is under compression, DBT reconstructs the breast tissue into thin slices. Viewing breast tissue in a 3D reconstructed set of thin images allows for the detection of abnormalities that may otherwise be obscured in a single flat image [3]. Benefits of DBT when compared to 2D mammography include improved cancer detection, higher sensitivity and specificity, reduced false positives, better performance in dense breast, and greater diagnostic confidence by radiologists [3]. Many institutions and hospitals routinely perform screening examinations with DBT, while others reserve it for diagnostic workup.

Localization

Radiologists describe the location of a lesion on breast mammography using a combination of clockface notation, quadrants, depth (anterior, middle, and posterior), and sometimes distance from the nipple or other reference points (Fig. 3.2) [4]. This detailed system of localization helps ensure that findings are clearly communicated and understood by all members of the healthcare team, and is critical for follow-up imaging, biopsy, or surgical planning.

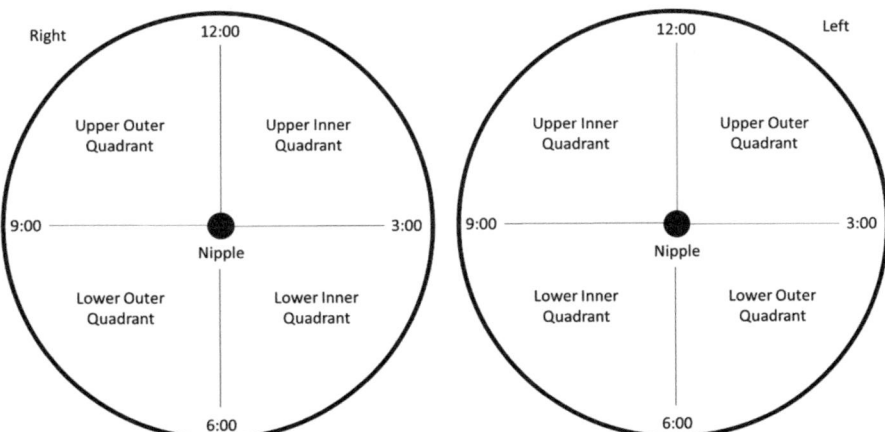

Fig. 3.2 This diagram shows two circular anatomical representations of the right and left breast. This is known as the clockface diagram, in which the breast is divided into four quadrants and clock positions to describe localization of breast findings. Note that the right outer breast is labeled as 9:00, but the left outer breast is considered 3:00, given that the perspective is as if the viewer were facing the patient

Clockface Notation

The breast is divided into an imaginary clockface, with the nipple at the center. The clock method allows for a precise description of the lesion's location in relation to the nipple:

- *12 o'clock*: The top of the breast, toward the chest wall.
- *6 o'clock*: The bottom of the breast, near the inframammary fold.
- *3 o'clock*: The lateral or outer side of the left breast or the medial or inner side of the right breast.
- *9 o'clock*: The lateral or outer side of the right breast or the medial or inner side of the left breast.

Quadrants

The breast is often divided into four quadrants using two imaginary lines: one vertical and one horizontal, both passing through the nipple. This results in the following quadrants:

- *Upper outer quadrant (UOQ)*: The upper and outer portion of the breast, near the axilla.
- *Upper inner quadrant (UIQ)*: The upper and inner portion of the breast, closer to the sternum.
- *Lower outer quadrant (LOQ)*: The lower and outer portion of the breast, near the inframammary fold.
- *Lower inner quadrant (LIQ)*: The lower and inner portion of the breast, near the chest wall and sternum.

Mean Glandular Dose

The mean glandular dose (MGD) is a measure of the radiation dose absorbed by the glandular tissue of the breast during a mammogram. It is the most relevant metric for assessing radiation risk in mammography because the glandular tissue is the most radiosensitive part of the breast. Factors that affect the MGD in a screening mammography are breast composition, breast thickness, X-ray beam energy, and compression. The mean glandular dose from a screening mammogram is 3 mGy [5, 6].

Breast Composition

Breast composition is noted on all mammography reports (Figs. 3.1 and 3.3). It describes the amount of fibroglandular tissue relative to fatty tissue [4]:

A: Almost entirely fatty
B: Scattered areas of fibroglandular density
C: Heterogeneously dense, which may obscure small masses
D: Extremely dense, which lowers the sensitivity of mammography

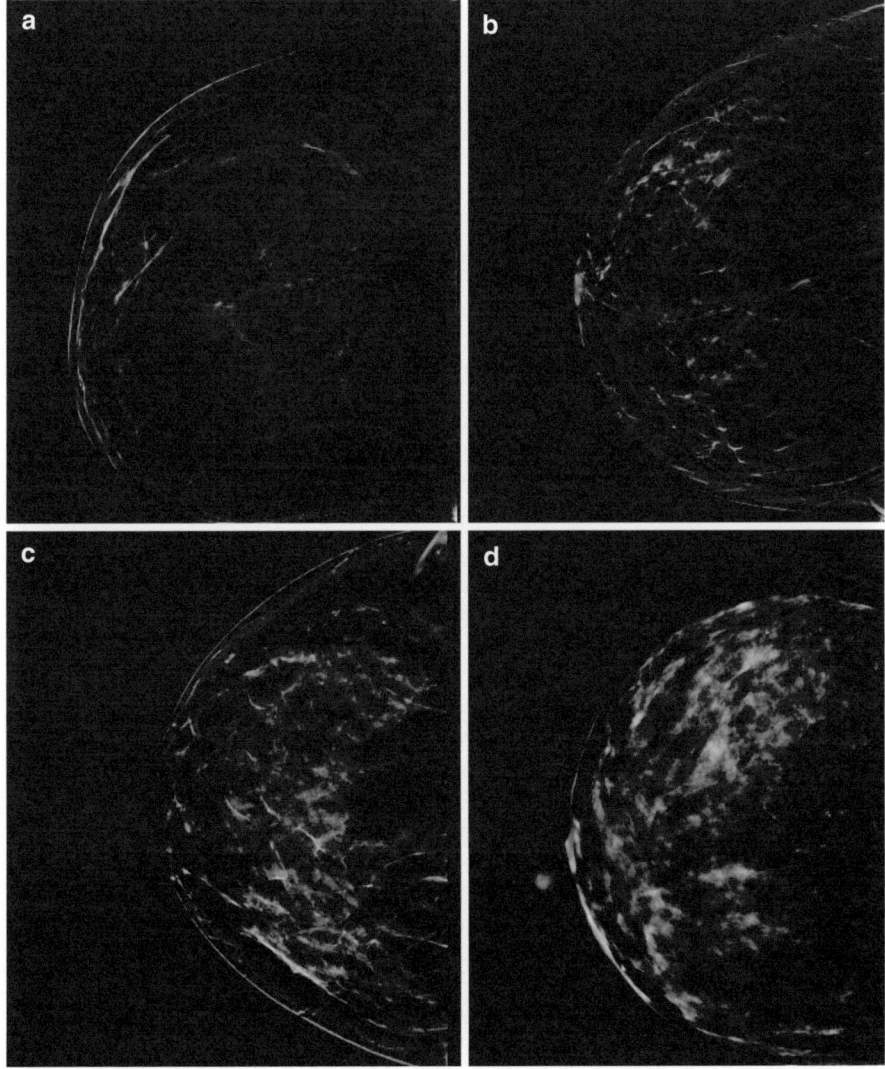

Fig. 3.3 Craniocaudal (CC) mammographic views demonstrate different breast density composition categories: (**a**) almost entirely fatty, (**b**) scattered areas of fibroglandular density, (**c**) heterogeneously dense, which may obscure small masses, (**d**) extremely dense, which lowers the sensitivity of mammography

Women with heterogeneously or extremely dense breasts have a slight increased risk of breast cancer by four to six times that of non-dense breasts [7–9]. The sensitivity of detecting findings on mammography decreases from approximately 85% in non-dense breasts to 60–80% in dense breasts [10, 11].

Breast Imaging-Reporting and Data System (BI-RADS®) for Screening Mammography

The Breast Imaging-Reporting and Data System (BI-RADS®) lexicon is a standardized system for categorizing findings on breast imaging studies to guide clinical decision-making and management. The BI-RADS® categories relevant for screening mammography include the following [4]:

BI-RADS® category	Description	Findings	Management recommendation
BI-RADS 0	Incomplete	Additional imaging or prior studies needed to complete the evaluation No definitive findings	Further imaging (e.g., additional mammographic views, ultrasound, or prior comparison) No definitive diagnosis until evaluation is complete
BI-RADS 1	Negative	No abnormal findings (e.g., masses, calcifications, architectural distortions) Normal breast tissue patterns	Routine screening follow-up (typically annual mammography)
BI-RADS 2	Benign	Benign findings such as: 　Simple cysts 　Fibroadenomas 　Intramammary lymph nodes 　Calcifications typical of benign processes	Routine screening follow-up (no further workup needed).

Recommendations for Screening

Screening recommendations for breast cancer vary depending on the overall lifetime risk of developing breast cancer. Multiple models exist for determining a woman's risk. These take into account various factors such as patient age, height, weight, family history, parity, menopausal status, exogenous hormone history, and additional factors such as genetic testing results if available and additional cancer history. The American College of Radiology and Society of Breast Imaging recommend all women undergoing risk assessment by the age of 30 [2]. Patients with a risk similar to the general population are deemed to have an average lifetime risk of developing breast cancer at 12.8% (1 in 8 women). Patients with a risk higher than or equal to 20% are deemed to have a high lifetime risk of developing breast cancer [2], and have additional screening recommendations.

Screening for Average Risk Patients

For average risk patients, the American College of Radiology and Society of Breast Imaging recommend screening start with annual screening mammograms at 40 years of age. By starting at age 40, there is approximately a 40% decrease in mortality from breast cancer [1]. There is no upper age limit for screening, unless severe comorbidities limit ability to obtain treatment or limit life expectancy. Screening mammography is not contraindicated in pregnancy, although controversy exists in the literature, and not contraindicated in lactation [12].

Screening for High-Risk Patients

For patients with a high lifetime risk of developing breast cancer, greater than or equal to 20%, the American College of Radiology and Society of Breast Imaging recommend earlier screening with mammography along with supplemental screening. Populations at high risk include, but are not limited to, patients with a family history of breast cancer, personal history of breast cancer or high-risk lesions, genetic mutation carriers, patients who have undergone chest radiation at a young age, minority populations, and those with higher breast density [2].

High-risk population	ACR screening recommendations for starting age, 2023[a]
Calculated lifetime risk of ≥20%	Annual DM ± DBT (age 40) Annual MRI (age 30)
Personal history of breast cancer before age 40	Annual DM ± DBT (age 40) Annual MRI if diagnosed before age 50 or dense breasts, or annual MRI can be considered from age of diagnosis
History of high-risk lesions diagnosed before age 40	Annual DM ± DBT (age 40) Consider annual MRI if other risk factors from age of diagnosis
Genetic mutation carriers or untested first-degree relatives	Annual DM ± DBT (age 40 if annual MRI, age 30 if not) Annual MRI (age 25–30)
History of chest/upper abdominal radiation at a young age	Annual DM ± DBT (age 40) Annual MRI (age 25 or 8 years after treatment, whichever is later)
Dense breast tissue	Annual DM ± DBT (age 40) Annual MRI or consider CEM or ultrasound as alternative to MRI (age 40 or earlier if other risk factors)

[a]Adapted from Monticciolio et al. [2]

Screening Breast MRI

Bilateral breast MRI with IV gadolinium contrast is the recommended supplemental screening tool as it has a higher sensitivity than mammography, ultrasound, or the combination of both, especially in higher risk patients [2]. By including a greater field of view, it also allows for evaluation of the chest wall, axillary, and internal mammary lymph nodes. Extra-mammary findings noted on breast MRI may include limited evaluation of the anterior lung fields and the upper abdomen. Breast MRI is contraindicated in pregnancy due to the IV gadolinium contrast, but not during lactation [12].

Breast MRI is performed with the patient lying prone in an MRI machine with a specialized breast coil. Images are obtained both before and after contrast administration. Contrast allows for physiologic evaluation of metabolically active tissues, including tumors that readily uptake the contrast due to angiogenesis, the development of leaky feeding blood vessels. Consecutive post-contrast image series are performed, including at 60–90 s after administration, when tumors often exhibit peak enhancement, and more delayed 5–7 min sequences for kinetic analysis [13]. Kinetic time-signal intensity curves evaluate the time it takes for contrast material to be removed from lesions. Using this, lesions can be categorized from least to most suspicious progressive, plateau, or washout kinetics (Fig. 3.4). Kinetic data supports the decision-making process, although morphology of a questioned lesion outweighs kinetic data. Many, although not all, tumors demonstrate rapid washout kinetics.

Emerging Potential Screening Modalities

Contrast-Enhanced Mammography (CEM)

Contrast-enhanced mammography (CEM) is a dual-energy 2D mammography technique performed utilizing IV iodinated contrast administration with mammography [14]. This allows for evaluation of morphology, similar to mammography, and physiology, similar to MRI [2, 15]. Two sets of images are evaluated: A low-energy image similar to 2D mammography; and a recombined contrast-enhanced image, in which non-enhancing breast parenchyma is no longer apparent, leaving enhancing tissues remaining for evaluation. CEM is currently being researched in multicenter trials to serve as a possible supplemental screening tool [16], especially for women at intermediate risk, between average risk of 12.8% and high risk of 20%. CEM is contraindicated in pregnancy, but not during lactation [12].

3 Screening and Diagnostic Imaging

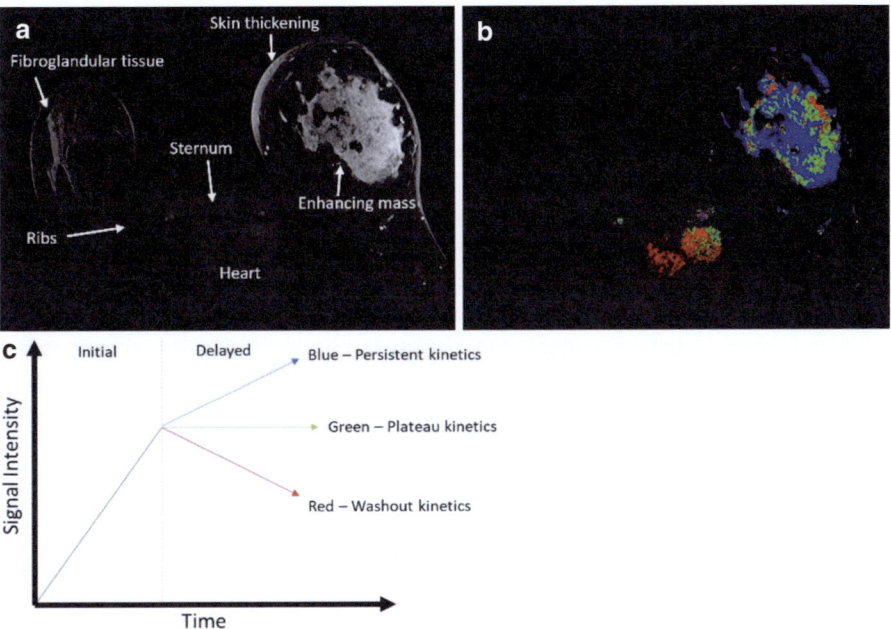

Fig. 3.4 Breast MRI of a 24-year-old patient with poorly differentiated invasive carcinoma of the left breast. (**a**) T1 post-contrast image demonstrates an irregular enhancing mass involving the majority of the left breast, along with left breast skin thickening. (**b**) T1 subtraction image with kinetic data shows the mass has mixed persistent, plateau and washout kinetics. (**c**) Kinetics curve showing the three types of enhancement that breast tissue may demonstrate, which are typically color-coded as blue for persistent, green for plateau, and red for washout delayed kinetics

Molecular Breast Imaging (MBI) or Breast-Specific Gamma Imaging (BSGI)

Molecular breast imaging (MBI) or breast-specific gamma imaging (BSGI) uses nuclear medicine to image the breasts for metabolically active tissue. A woman undergoes intravenous injection of technetium-99m sestamibi (^{99m}Tc-sestamibi), a radioisotope bound to a protein molecule that accumulates in mitochondria in metabolically active cells [17]. Administration of as low as 8mCI of Tc-99m are thought to be sufficient, but the standard dosage is 20–30 mCi [17]. Standard CC and MLO views of each breast are acquired by a gamma camera for 5–10 min [17]. As cancer cells are generally metabolically active, this can serve as a supplemental screening method for women at high risk. However, MBI does not provide detailed morphologic data, involves whole-body radiation exposures, and has a long examination time of up to 40 min, which limits its use. MBI is also contraindicated in pregnancy.

Diagnostic Breast Imaging

Diagnostic Mammography

Indications

Diagnostic breast mammography is used to evaluate specific breast concerns or abnormalities. Indications for diagnostic mammography and possible targeted ultrasound include abnormal findings on screening mammography (such as masses, asymmetries, architectural distortion or suspicious calcifications), symptoms or clinical concerns (such as palpable lumps or masses, nipple changes, skin changes, or focal breast pain), follow-up of previously detected abnormalities, and staging and monitoring treatment response of known cancer [18]. Diagnostic mammography is performed in real-time with an interpreting radiologist present.

A standardized BI-RADS lexicon ensures consistency in reporting findings and aids in determining the level of suspicion for breast cancer [4]. The lexicon includes descriptions of breast composition, masses, calcifications, asymmetries, architectural distortion, and associated features (Figs. 3.5, 3.6, 3.7, and 3.8).

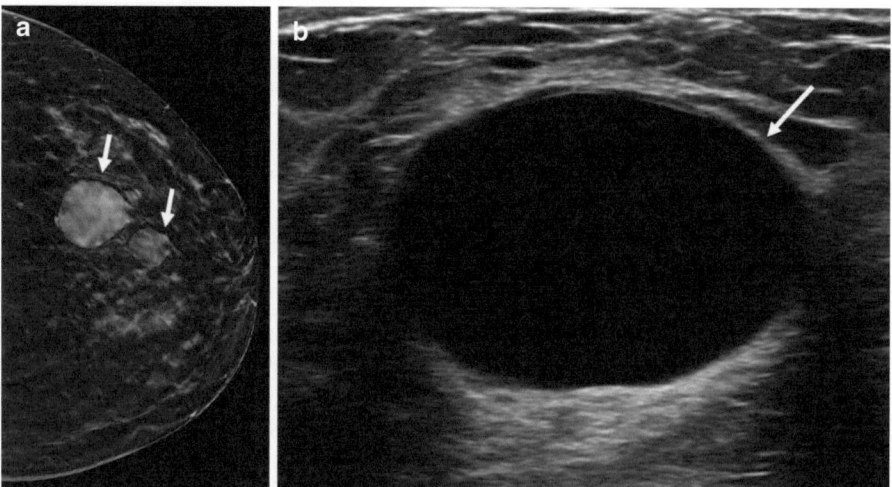

Fig. 3.5 (**a**) Craniocaudal tomosynthesis image of the left breast showing two adjacent oval, equal density masses with circumscribed margins (arrows). (**b**) Ultrasound of the left breast performed in the same patient shows an oval anechoic mass with circumscribed margins and posterior acoustic shadowing consistent with a simple cyst (arrow), corresponding to one of the mammographic findings

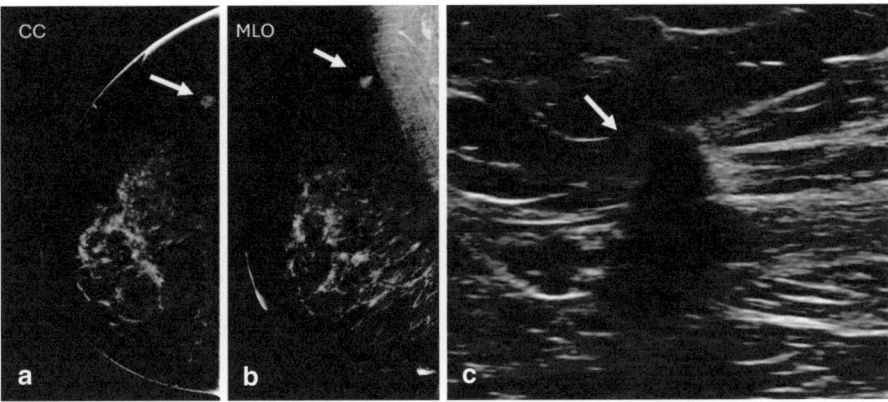

Fig. 3.6 A 55-year-old patient with right breast cancer presenting as an irregular mass. (**a, b**) Craniocaudal and mediolateral oblique mammographic views of the right breast show an irregular mass with spiculated margins in the right upper outer posterior breast (arrows). (**c**) Ultrasound of the right breast performed in the same patient shows an irregular, hypoechoic, anti-parallel mass with spiculated margins and an echogenic halo corresponding to the mammographic mass (arrow). This was biopsied with pathology consistent with invasive ductal carcinoma

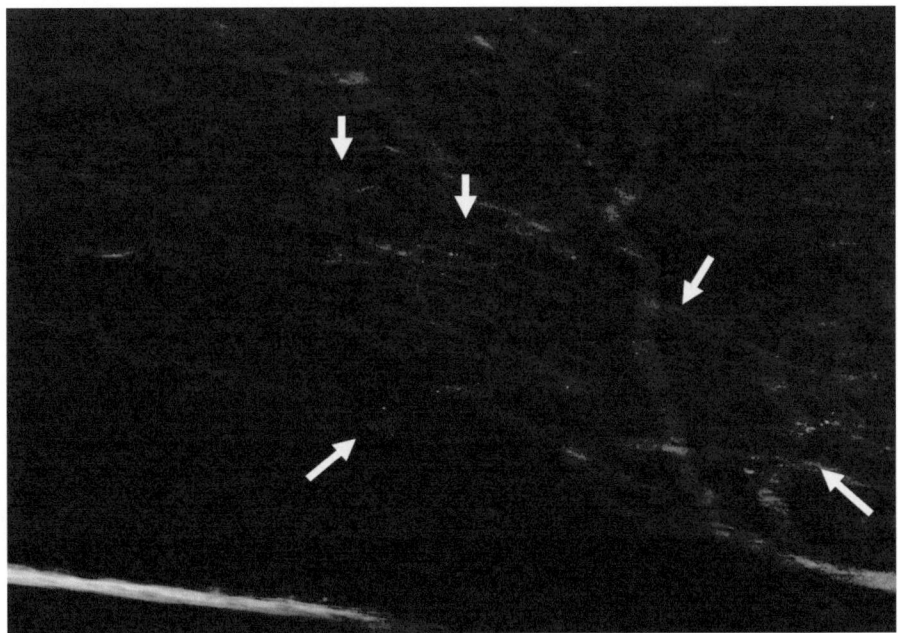

Fig. 3.7 A 68-year-old patient with right breast cancer presenting as calcifications. Spot magnification craniocaudal view demonstrates right inner breast posterior depth segmental fine pleomorphic calcifications (arrows). Biopsy of the calcifications revealed ductal carcinoma in situ (DCIS)

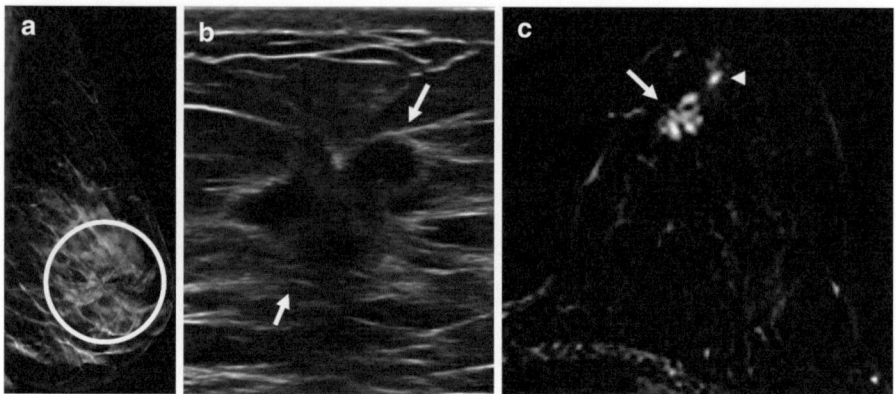

Fig. 3.8 A 51-year-old patient with left breast cancer. (**a**) Mediolateral tomosynthesis view demonstrates an architectural distortion in the central breast (circled). (**b**) Ultrasound shows a hypoechoic irregular mass with spiculated margins in the upper inner breast (arrow). (**c**) Axial subtracted T1 post-contrast MRI shows a heterogeneously enhancing irregular mass with spiculated margins (arrow) and an adjacent satellite mass (arrowhead)

Mass

A mass is defined as a three-dimensional lesion that occupies space and is distinguishable from surrounding tissue. The lexicon describes defining characteristics of shape, parallel or non-parallel orientation, margin, echogenicity, and posterior acoustic features.

Shape:
- Round: Spherical or ball-like.
- Oval: Elliptical or egg-shaped.
- Irregular: Non-uniform shape.

Margins:
- Circumscribed: Well-defined and sharp edges. Considered when >75% of the lesion is defined.
- Obscured: Partially hidden by overlapping tissue.
- Microlobulated: Small lobulations (>3) on the margin.
- Indistinct: Poorly defined (suspicious).
- Spiculated: Radiating lines from the margin (highly suspicious).

Density:
- Fat-containing: Indicates benign lesions like lipomas or oil cysts.
- Low density: Less dense than surrounding tissue.
- Equal density: Same as surrounding tissue.
- High density: Denser than surrounding tissue.

Types of Calcifications in Breast Mammography

Calcifications are tiny deposits of calcium that appear as hyperdense (white spots) on a mammogram. They are categorized based on their morphology and distribution. Understanding the type of calcifications helps to differentiate between benign and potentially malignant findings.

Benign Calcifications

Benign calcifications are typically harmless and do not require further investigation. Common types include the following:

Type	Description	Examples
Skin (dermal)	Well-defined, ring-like, or hollow/lucent calcifications often associated with sweat glands or skin lesions	Dermal calcifications from sebaceous cysts or scarring
Vascular	Linear or parallel "railroad track" calcifications following blood vessels	Arterial calcifications (common in older women or those with vascular disease)
Coarse	Large, irregular, or chunky calcifications	Associated with involuting fibroadenomas
Large rod-like	Thick, linear, rod-like calcifications with tram-track or branching appearance	Associated with duct ectasia (dilatation of milk ducts), typically in postmenopausal women. Also known as plasma cell mastitis
Round	Small, uniform, well-circumscribed calcifications (<1 mm in size)	Found in benign lesions or scattered in normal breast tissue. May be considered probably benign if grouped and without priors. May be considered suspicious if new from priors and/or in a concerning pattern of distribution
Rim	Thin, smooth, circular, or oval calcifications that outline a structure	Associated with oil cysts (due to fat necrosis)
Dystrophic	Irregular, fragmented, or "cheese-like" calcifications in areas of prior trauma, surgery, or radiation	Post-surgical or post-radiation changes
Milk of calcium	Layering or "teacup-shaped" calcifications seen on lateral views	Found in cysts or dilated ducts
Suture	Linear or beaded calcifications	Follow the path of a surgical suture

Suspicious Calcifications

Calcifications that may indicate a level of suspicion for malignancy include the following:

Type	Description	Significance
Amorphous	Calcifications with no clearly defined shape or form Appear as indistinct, fuzzy, or powdery deposits	Considered intermediate suspicion for malignancy but not definitively benign May be associated with benign processes such as fibrocystic changes, columnar cell changes, or low-grade ductal carcinoma in situ (DCIS)
Course heterogeneous	Calcifications that are irregular, larger than 0.5 mm, and vary in size and shape Appears denser than amorphous calcifications but lack fine detail	Considered intermediate suspicion for malignancy Associated with benign conditions (e.g., fibrocystic changes or fat necrosis) or low- to intermediate-grade DCIS
Fine pleomorphic	Tiny, irregularly shaped calcifications of varying sizes and shapes Appear as fine, granular deposits with no uniformity	Considered high suspicion for malignancy Frequently associated with high-grade DCIS or invasive carcinoma
Fine linear or fine-linear branching	Thin, linear, or branching calcifications that resemble casts of ducts Often irregular and discontinuous, with a "branching" appearance	Considered the highest suspicion for malignancy Strongly associated with high-grade DCIS, and invasive ductal carcinoma

Distribution Patterns

The distribution of calcifications can help determine their significance and level of suspicion:

Pattern	Description	Implications
Diffuse	Randomly distributed throughout the breast	Usually benign
Regional	In a large area of one quadrant	May be benign or malignant; requires evaluation
Grouped	Found in a small area (<2 cm)	Can be benign or malignant; morphology determines suspicion level
Linear	Along a ductal distribution	May be suspicious for malignancy (i.e., DCIS)
Segmental	Following the anatomy of a duct or segment	Suspicious for malignancy, especially if pleomorphic or linear calcifications

Architectural Distortion

An architectural distortion is an abnormal arrangement of breast tissue with no visible mass, presenting as radiating lines or focal retraction. It is often associated with malignancy but can also occur post-surgery, post-radiation, or with radial scars.

Asymmetries

Asymmetries are differences in density or architecture between breasts.

Types:
- *Asymmetry*: One-sided density without mass-like features.
- *Focal Asymmetry*: A localized asymmetry seen on two views.
- *Developing Asymmetry*: New or enlarging asymmetry (suspicious).
- *Global Asymmetry*: A larger region of one-sided density.

Supplemental Views

View	Description	Purpose	Technique
Mediolateral (ML)	A side-to-side view taken perpendicular to the CC view	Provides better visualization of certain lesions or areas not well seen in MLO	The breast is compressed horizontally, and the X-ray beam travels from the medial side to the lateral side
Lateromedial (LM)	The reverse of the ML view, with the beam traveling from lateral to medial	Useful for clarifying findings in the inner breast or evaluating suspected abnormalities	The breast is compressed at an angle (40–60°) between the plates. The X-ray beam travels from the outer (lateral) side to the inner (medial) side
Delayed	Images taken after a period of time to assess changes in breast findings	To observe how a lesion behaves over time to help differentiate benign from malignant findings Often used in LM or ML views to evaluate for layering calcifications	Take additional images at certain views at intervals after initial imaging

(continued)

View	Description	Purpose	Technique
Tangential	Focused views designed to image a specific area of concern in the breast, particularly lesions near the skin or palpable abnormalities	Assess palpable lumps, skin lesions, or clip markers	The X-ray beam is angled tangentially (parallel to the skin) to avoid overlap of deeper tissues
Rolled	Views in which the breast tissue is "rolled" in different directions during imaging to separate overlapping tissues	To distinguish between true lesions and artifacts caused by overlapping normal tissue Helps clarify an asymmetry seen in standard views, especially on CC view Used to confirm whether an abnormality persists after tissue is displaced	The breast is compressed as usual, and then the tissue is physically rolled in a specific direction: *Rolled medial (RM)*: Tissue is rolled toward the middle of the chest *Rolled lateral (RL)*: Tissue is rolled toward the outer side of the chest *Rolled superior (RS)*: Tissue is rolled upward *Rolled inferior (RI)*: Tissue is rolled downward
Spot compression	A close-up view of a specific area of the breast using focused compression	Improves detail and reduces overlapping tissues for better evaluation of abnormalities	Only the area of interest is compressed with a smaller paddle
Magnification	A magnified view of a specific region of the breast	Used to examine calcifications or small lesions more closely	A magnification platform is used to increase the distance between the breast and the image receptor
Cleavage	Focuses on the medial (inner) breast tissue close to the chest wall	Evaluates abnormalities located deep in the cleavage area	Both breasts are positioned together, and the X-ray is taken centrally

Diagnostic Ultrasound

Indications for diagnostic ultrasound are similar to that of mammography. Diagnostic ultrasound is used as the first-line imaging modality in women who are younger than 30 years of age. Diagnostic ultrasound often follows diagnostic mammography as a problem-solving tool, and is indicated when diagnostic mammography is negative in evaluation of clinical symptoms, including palpable areas of concern and focal (not diffuse) pain, nipple changes, or skin thickening [19].

There is a standardized BI-RADS lexicon used to describe sonographic findings in the breast [20]. Below is an overview of the key features described in the BI-RADS ultrasound lexicon (Figs. 3.5, 3.6, and 3.8).

Mass

A mass is defined as a three-dimensional lesion that occupies space and is distinguishable from surrounding tissue. The lexicon describes its shape, orientation, margin, echogenicity, and posterior acoustic features.

Shape
- Round: Spherical or nearly spherical.
- Oval: Elliptical lesions.
- Irregular: Non-uniform or asymmetric (suspicious).

Orientation
- Parallel: Long axis lies parallel to the skin (wider than tall).
- Not Parallel: Long axis is perpendicular to the skin (taller than wide; suspicious).

Margin
- Circumscribed: Well-defined and smooth.
- Indistinct: Poorly defined; blends with surrounding tissue.
- Angular: Sharp corners; suggests malignancy.
- Microlobulated: Small lobulations (>3) along the margin (suspicious).
- Spiculated: Radiating lines; strongly associated with malignancy.

Echogenicity
- Anechoic: Appears completely black (e.g., simple cysts).
- Hypoechoic: Darker than surrounding tissue.
- Isoechoic: Similar echogenicity to surrounding tissue.
- Hyperechoic: Brighter than surrounding tissue.
- Complex: Mixed echogenic and anechoic areas (e.g., complex cysts).

Posterior Acoustic Features
- No enhancement: No significant posterior feature.
- Enhancement: Increased brightness behind the mass (often benign).
- Shadowing: Reduced brightness behind the mass (may suggest malignancy).
- Mixed effects: Combination of shadowing and enhancement.

Calcifications

Calcifications on ultrasound are more challenging to detect compared to mammography. If seen, they are described as:

- *Macrocalcifications*: Coarse, large calcifications (often benign).
- *Microcalcifications*: Tiny, clustered calcifications (suspicious for malignancy).

Diagnostic MRI

Overview

Diagnostic MRI is indicated in specific scenarios and plays an important role in determining extent of disease in diagnosis and treatment of known breast cancer. MRI provides a wider field of view including the anterior chest, making it an invaluable tool for disease evaluation, including the chest wall and lymph node stations.

Indications

Problem-solving breast MRI is performed with and without IV gadolinium contrast for a variety of indications. These include indeterminate or equivocal diagnostic workup with mammography and ultrasound, suspicious nipple discharge (spontaneous unilateral bloody or serous nipple discharge), skin changes, or suspicious lesions that cannot be definitively imaged with other modalities or with discordant biopsy results requiring further evaluation [13].

In a patient with newly diagnosed breast cancer, a bilateral breast MRI can be used for staging and disease extent evaluation. In addition to evaluating lesions within the breast, MRI allows for further evaluation of potential skin thickening and edema; skin, nipple-areolar complex, and chest wall musculature enhancement that most likely indicates tumor involvement; level I, II, and III axillary lymph nodes, internal mammary lymph nodes, and anterior ribs and sternum. The obtained images also provide a cursory look at the anterior liver and lungs.

If the patient is undergoing neoadjuvant therapy, a contrast-enhanced bilateral breast MRI can be used for imaging evaluation of treatment response (Fig. 3.9) [21, 22]. By comparing pre- and post-neoadjuvant therapy MRIs, response can be determined, in part per the Response Evaluation Criteria in Solid Tumors (RECIST) guidelines [21, 23]. Complete response (CR) is defined as disappearance of all target lesions and normalization of lymph nodes. Partial response (PR) is defined as at least 30% decrease in the size of target lesions. Stable disease (SD) refers to insufficient shrinkage of target lesions or insufficient target lesion growth. Progressive disease (PD) is defined as at least 20% increase in size of target lesions, including at least an absolute increase of at least 5 mm. New lesions also constitute progressive

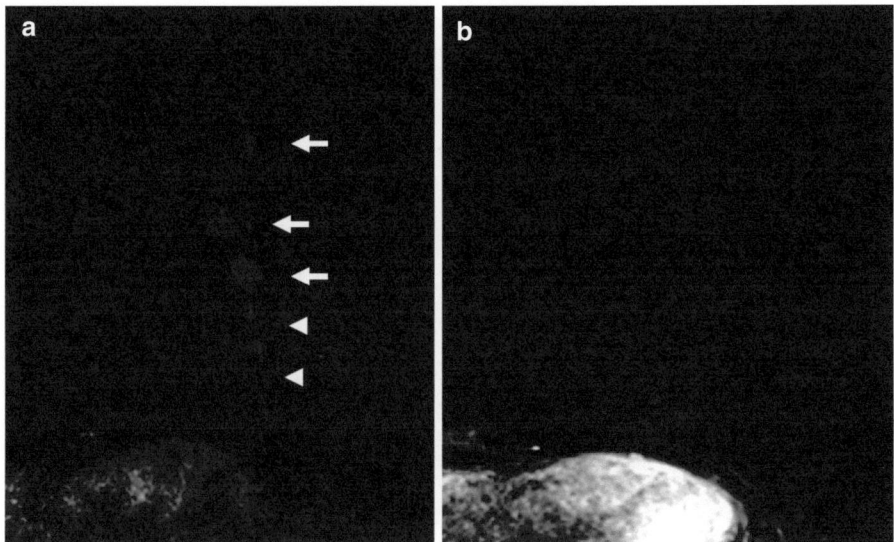

Fig. 3.9 A 38-year-old patient with multifocal left breast malignancy on neoadjuvant therapy on axial subtracted T1 post-contrast MRI. Before treatment (**a**), heterogeneously enhancing irregular masses (arrows) and posterior non-mass enhancement (arrowhead) is present throughout the lower outer breast. After (**b**) neoadjuvant therapy, the findings have resolved. This is categorized as a complete imaging response to treatment with no evidence of malignancy on the post-treatment imaging

disease [23]. RECIST does not apply to breast imaging as a whole, as the criteria excludes mammography and ultrasound and is not used for axillary lymph node evaluation, but is does provide some guidance. In practice, radiologists compare tumor size and MR enhancement patterns using BI-RADS® lexicon descriptors and loosely categorize response to therapy based upon the four categories of complete, partial, stable, or progressive [22].

A breast MRI without contrast is the best imaging modality to assess silicone implant integrity [24]. Specific sequences that accentuate fluid (T2-weighted images), silicone (silicone-weighted images), and the lack of silicone (silicone subtraction images) can help assess for implant compromise including peri-implant fluid, capsular integrity, and intra- and extra-capsular rupture. Intravenous gadolinium contrast is not administered for these exams, and as such the evaluation for malignancy is limited (Fig. 3.10).

Currently, breast MRI is not specifically indicated for surveillance in patients who have undergone mastectomy. However, MRI can provide valuable information about the reconstructed breast, chest wall, and axilla and may be added as an additional imaging modality for problem-solving in these patients.

There is a standardized BI-RADS lexicon used to describe MRI findings in the breast [25].

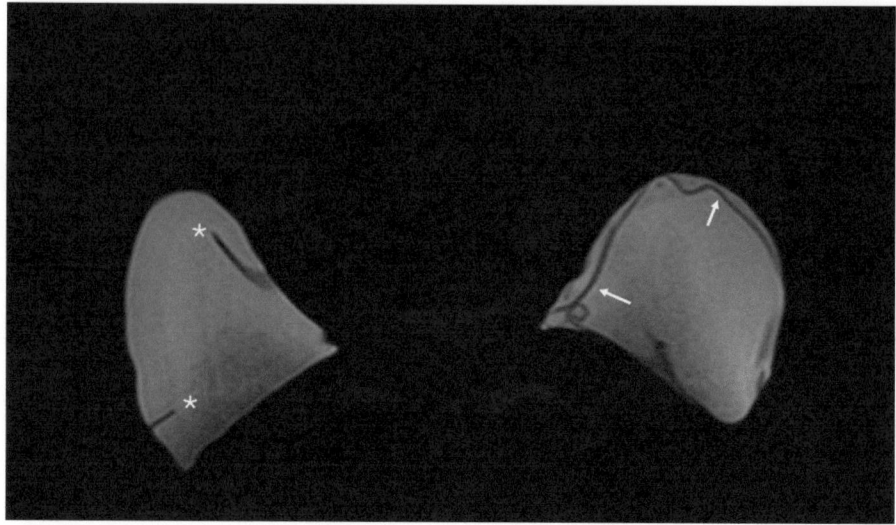

Fig. 3.10 Non-contrast bilateral breast MRI performed to assess for silicone implant integrity. Bilateral retropectoral silicone implants. The right implant demonstrated normal axial folds (*) without evidence of rupture. The left implant demonstrates multiple curvilinear lines floating in silicone (arrows), known as the "linguini sign," indicating intracapsular rupture

Diagnostic Contrast-Enhanced Mammography

CEM is the newest emerging breast imaging modality and deemed appropriate for use in the diagnostic setting, approved by the FDA in 2011 [14]. It can be used similar to mammography for problem solving, extent of disease workup, and neoadjuvant therapy response assessment. It can also be considered for patients who may not be a candidate for MRI. A standardized BI-RADS lexicon for CEM was published in 2022 [15].

Breast Imaging-Reporting and Data System (BI-RADS®) for Diagnostic Imaging

The Breast Imaging-Reporting and Data System is a standardized system for categorizing findings on breast imaging studies to guide clinical decision-making and management. The BI-RADS® categories relevant for diagnostic mammography, ultrasound, and MRI include the following:

BI-RADS category	Description	Findings	Management recommendation
BI-RADS 0	Incomplete	Additional imaging or prior studies needed to complete the evaluation	No definitive diagnosis until evaluation is complete This is rarely used in diagnostic imaging as next steps in management are typically provided, but may be helpful in certain circumstances
BI-RADS 1	Negative	No abnormal findings (e.g., masses, calcifications, architectural distortions) Normal breast tissue patterns	Routine screening follow-up (typically annual mammography)

BI-RADS 2	Benign	Benign findings such as:
		  Simple cysts
		  Fibroadenomas
		  Intramammary lymph nodes
		  Calcifications typical of benign processes
			Routine screening follow-up (no further workup needed)

BI-RADS 3	Probably benign	Defined as a likelihood of malignancy between 0% and 2% Includes oval, circumscribed masses; grouped round calcifications; nonpalpable asymmetries on a baseline mammogram Includes complicated cysts and groups of clustered microcysts MRI is not yet defined, but often includes findings associated with T2 hyperintensity, including masses, non-mass enhancement, and foci [26]	Follow-up imaging over a 2-year time frame to assess stability. If the finding does not change over 2 years or is less conspicuous, it is deemed benign. If there is any indication of suspicious features or growth, the finding is re-categorized After initial diagnostic evaluation, the patient returns at 6-months → 6-months → 1 year to complete the 2-year cycle

BI-RADS 4	Suspicious	Defined as >2% but ≤95% chance of malignancy
		Sometimes categorized further:
		  4A (low): >2% but ≤10%
		  4B (moderate): >10% but ≤50%
		  4C (high): >50% but ≤95%
			Requires tissue diagnosis

BI-RADS 5	Highly suspicious	Defined as ≥95% chance of malignancy	Requires tissue diagnosis
BI-RADS 6	Biopsy-proven malignancy	Known breast cancer Used for exams after proof of malignancy and no other abnormalities, including for extent of disease that does not require further biopsies or neoadjuvant treatment response	Appropriate oncologic and surgical management

Biopsy Modalities

Once a finding is deemed suspicious on diagnostic imaging (BI-RADS 4 or 5), tissue confirmation is recommended with biopsy. Biopsies can be performed under ultrasound, mammography and/or tomosynthesis, and MRI guidance, and most recently CEM. Choosing the proper biopsy modality is based upon multiple factors, including on which modality the finding is best visualized, the safety and efficacy of the approach, and patient factors of age, ease of positioning, and comfort. Ultrasound is often the first method of choice if a target is clearly visualized, as it is widely available and easiest for the patient, with low propensity for vasovagal reactions. Stereotactic (mammogram)-guided biopsies are often used for calcifications or mammogram-only detected findings. Breast MRI biopsies are used for MRI-only detected findings.

Two types of tissue sampling are available: core needle biopsy and fine needle aspiration. Core needle biopsy is performed with biopsy devices in sizes ranging from 18 gauge to 9 gauge, and can be done with or without vacuum assistance and with each modality (ultrasound, stereotactic/mammogram guidance, and MRI). A metal biopsy marker clip is placed post-procedure, which comes in many different formulations and shapes and allows for verification of targeting and follow-up and removal of the lesion if necessary. Specimen cores are sent to pathology for evaluation.

Ultrasound-guided fine needle aspiration is performed with needle sizes ranging from 20 to 25 gauge, and is predominantly performed for sampling of axillary lymph nodes. Cytology to detect malignancy or flow cytometry to detect lymphoproliferative disease can be performed. Special uses of fine needle aspiration also include, but are not limited to, technically challenging locations near implants or in post-mastectomy patients. Ultrasound-guided aspiration can also be performed of cystic lesions in the breast, after which the aspirate can be discarded, or if bloody, sent for cytologic evaluation. Abscess drainages can be performed and sent for microbiology evaluation.

Common procedure risks including bleeding, bruising, pain, and infection, which are mitigated by appropriate compression maneuvers, sterile technique, and post-procedure care. The extent of post-procedure care varies based on needle size and biopsy type. A fine needle or cyst aspiration requires minimal care with a small bandage placed at the entry site and no restrictions. Common post-core needle biopsy restrictions include lifting restrictions on the biopsied side for approximately 48–72 h and no submerging the affected area in water for approximately 1 week. Over-the-counter acetaminophen and on-and-off cold ice pack compresses are often enough to control any minimal discomfort the patient may experience afterwards.

Conclusion

Breast imaging radiologists provide a critical service to the care of women with benign breast disease and breast cancer. Preventative routine annual screening mammography reduces breast cancer mortality by at least 40% [1, 2]. Screening for high-risk patients is performed with the use of annual contrast-enhanced breast MRI in addition to mammography. Additional emerging modalities of CEM and MBI may play a future role in transforming screening as personalized management for intermediate risk patients unfolds. Diagnostic imaging with mammogram, ultrasound, MRI, and most recently CEM, is essential for appropriate management of benign and malignant conditions. It is important to have a mastery of fundamentals of breast imaging, including BI-RADS. Whether it be in preventative screening measures or in diagnostic workup, breast imaging radiologists are a key component of the multidisciplinary team, interacting with medical assistant and technologist staff, referring providers, breast surgeons, breast oncologists, and radiation oncologists to provide comprehensive care together.

References

1. Monticciolo DL, Malak SF, Friedewald SM, Eby PR, Newell MS, Moy L, et al. Breast cancer screening recommendations inclusive of all women at average risk: update from the ACR and Society of Breast Imaging. J Am Coll Radiol. 2021;18(9):1280–8.
2. Monticciolo DL, Newell MS, Moy L, Lee CS, Destounis SV. Breast cancer screening for women at higher-than-average risk: updated recommendations from the ACR. J Am Coll Radiol. 2023;20(9):902–14.
3. Butler R, Conant EF, Philpotts L. Digital breast tomosynthesis: what have we learned? J Breast Imaging. 2019;1(1):9–22.
4. Sickles EA, D'Orsi CJ, Bassett LW, et al. ACR BI-RADS® mammography. In: ACR BI-RADS® atlas, breast imaging reporting and data system. Reston: American College of Radiology; 2013.
5. Hendrick RE. Radiation doses and risks in breast screening. J Breast Imaging. 2020;2(3):188–200.
6. Sanders JW, Pavlicek W, Stefan W, Hanson J, Sharpe RE, Patel BK. Digital mammography, tomosynthesis, and contrast-enhanced mammography: intraindividual comparison of mean glandular dose for screening examinations. Am J Roentgenol. 2025;224(3):e2432150. Available from: https://ajronline.org/doi/10.2214/AJR.24.32150.
7. Boyd NF, Martin LJ, Bronskill M, Yaffe MJ, Duric N, Minkin S. Breast tissue composition and susceptibility to breast cancer. JNCI J Natl Cancer Inst. 2010;102(16):1224–37.
8. Boyd NF, Guo H, Martin LJ, Sun L, Stone J, Fishell E, et al. Mammographic density and the risk and detection of breast cancer. N Engl J Med. 2007;356(3):227–36.
9. Park B, Cho HM, Lee EH, Song S, Suh M, Choi KS, et al. Does breast density measured through population-based screening independently increase breast cancer risk in Asian females? Clin Epidemiol. 2018;10:61–70.

10. Freer PE. Mammographic breast density: impact on breast cancer risk and implications for screening. Radiographics. 2015;35(2):302–15.
11. Winkler NS, Raza S, Mackesy M, Birdwell RL. Breast density: clinical implications and assessment methods. Radiographics. 2015;35(2):316–24.
12. Portnow LH, Snider LC, Bolivar KE, Bychkovsky BL, Klehm MR, Yeh ED, et al. Breast cancer screening in high-risk women during pregnancy and lactation. J Breast Imaging. 2023;5(5):508–19.
13. Mann RM, Cho N, Moy L. Breast MRI: state of the art. Radiology. 2019;292(3):520–36.
14. Jochelson MS, Lobbes MBI. Contrast-enhanced mammography: state of the art. Radiology. 2021;299(1):36–48.
15. Lee CH, Phillips J, Sung JS, Lewin JM, Newell MS. ACR BI-RADS® contrast enhanced mammography (CEM). In: ACR BI-RADS® atlas, breast imaging reporting and data system. Reston: American College of Radiology; 2022.
16. Coffey K, Jochelson MS. Contrast-enhanced mammography in breast cancer screening. Eur J Radiol. 2022;156:110513. Available from: https://www.ejradiology.com/article/S0720-048X(22)00363-1/fulltext.
17. American College of Radiology. ACR practice parameter for the performance of molecular breast imaging (MBI) using a dedicated gamma camera. 2022 [Internet]. [cited 2025 Jan 27]. Available from: https://gravitas.acr.org/PPTS/GetDocumentView?docId=144+&releaseId=2.
18. American College of Radiology. ACR practice parameter for the performance of screening and diagnostic mammography. 2023 [Internet]. [cited 2025 Jan 31]. Available from: https://gravitas.acr.org/PPTS/GetDocumentView?docId=8+&releaseId=2.
19. American College of Radiology. ACR practice parameter for the performance of diagnostic breast ultrasound examination. 2021 [Internet]. [cited 2025 Jan 31]. Available from: https://gravitas.acr.org/PPTS/GetDocumentView?docId=124+&releaseId=2.
20. Mendelson EB, Böhm-Vélez M, Berg WA, et al. ACR BI-RADS® ultrasound. In: ACR BI-RADS® atlas, breast imaging reporting and data system. Reston: American College of Radiology; 2013.
21. Reig B, Lewin AA, Du L, Heacock L, Toth HK, Heller SL, et al. Breast MRI for evaluation of response to neoadjuvant therapy. Radiographics. 2021;41(3):665–79.
22. Fowler AM, Mankoff DA, Joe BN. Imaging neoadjuvant therapy response in breast cancer. Radiology. 2017;285(2):358–75.
23. Eisenhauer EA, Therasse P, Bogaerts J, Schwartz LH, Sargent D, Ford R, et al. New response evaluation criteria in solid tumours: revised RECIST guideline (version 1.1). Eur J Cancer. 2009;45(2):228–47.
24. Chetlen A, Niell BL, Brown A, Baskies AM, Battaglia T, Chen A, et al. ACR appropriateness criteria® breast implant evaluation: 2023 update. J Am Coll Radiol. 2023;20(11):S329–50.
25. Morris EA, Comstock CE, Lee CH, et al. ACR BI-RADS® magnetic resonance imaging. In: ACR BI-RADS® atlas, breast imaging reporting and data system. Reston: American College of Radiology; 2013.
26. Fazeli S, Stepenosky J, Guirguis MS, Adrada B, Rakow-Penner R, Ojeda-Fournier H. Understanding BI-RADS category 3. Radiographics. 2025;45(1):e240169.

Chapter 4
Surgical Treatment of Breast Cancer

Claire Morton and Christina Minami

Introduction

Breast cancer remains the most commonly diagnosed cancer among women in the United States [1]. As a result of robust screening, most women are fortunately diagnosed in early stages of disease. Patients without metastatic disease are generally treated with surgical intervention, along with systemic therapies (including chemotherapy, immunotherapy, and endocrine therapy) and, in certain cases, radiation. Surgery can be accompanied by reconstructive procedures, such as oncoplastic procedures in breast-conserving cases and implant-based or autologous tissue reconstruction after mastectomy [2]. A number of techniques for surgical management of early-stage breast cancer are available and can be employed based on extent of disease and patient preference. Clear physician-patient communication regarding surgical options and their associated risks and benefits is pivotal to helping breast cancer patients make treatment choices that are knowledgeable and consistent with their values.

C. Morton
Center for Surgery and Public Health, Brigham and Women's Hospital, Department of Surgery, Yale New Haven Hospital, New Haven, CT, USA

C. Minami (✉)
Department of Surgery, Brigham and Women's Hospital, Breast Oncology Program, Dana-Farber/Brigham Cancer Center, Boston, MA, USA
e-mail: cminami@mgb.org

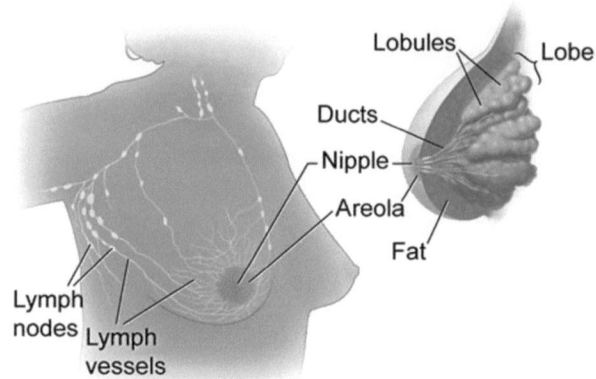

Fig. 4.1 Image credited to the National Cancer Institute Visuals Online, Don Bliss (Illustrator)

Anatomy of the Breast (Fig. 4.1)

Anatomic Boundaries of the Breast

Medial: lateral border of the sternum
Lateral: anterior border of the latissimus dorsi
Superior: clavicle
Inferior: insertion of the rectus abdominis
Posterior: chest wall (2/3 overlying the pectoralis major, 1/3 overlying the serratus anterior and upper portion of the oblique)
Anterior: skin

The "tail of Spence" includes breast tissue which extends into the axilla [3].

The breast is often described in quadrants: upper/lower (or superior/inferior) and inner/outer (or medial/lateral), from the patient's perspective, or as a clock face, from the observer's perspective (e.g., 2 o'clock on the left breast would be found in the upper outer or superior lateral quadrant). Lateral and anterior cutaneous branches of the second through sixth intercostal nerve provide major sensory innervation to the breast.

Blood Supply

The medial and central portions of the breast receive blood from the anterior perforating intercostal arteries which in turn arise from the internal thoracic/internal mammary artery. The remainder of the blood supply to the breast originates from branches of the lateral thoracic artery, pectoral branches of the thoracoacromial artery, and branches of the posterior intercostal arteries. The venous supply drains toward the axilla via the perforating branches of the internal thoracic vein, posterior intercostal vein, and tributaries of the axillary vein [4]. Batson's plexus is a valveless venous plexus that allows for direct bony metastasis of breast cancer to the spine.

Axillary Lymph Nodes

The majority of the lymphatic drainage of the breast occurs via the axilla. Medial aspects of the breast may drain to the internal mammary nodes, but routine excision of internal mammary nodes is no longer pursued given the risk/benefit ratio.

Anatomic Boundaries of the Axilla

Superior: axillary vein
Inferior: no clear inferior anatomic border exists
Medial: see below—typical axillary lymph node dissections for breast cancer include Levels I and II
Lateral: border of the latissimus dorsi
Anterior: clavipectoral fascia
Posterior: subscapularis muscle

Levels of Axillary Lymph Nodes:

Level I: lateral to pectoralis minor muscle
Level II: deep to the pectoralis minor

Note: Rotter's nodes (nodes between the pectoralis major and minor) are not routinely excised during axillary lymph node dissections.

Level III: medial to pectoralis minor muscle

Nerves and Potential Effects of Nerve Injury in the Axilla

- Long thoracic nerve: innervates the serratus anterior.
  (a) Injury presents as winging of the scapula, shoulder pain, and inability to raise the arm above shoulder level.

- Thoracodorsal nerve: innervates the latissimus dorsi.
    (a) Injury presents as weakened arm pull-ups and adduction.
- Medial pectoral nerve: innervates both the pectoralis major and the pectoralis minor.
    (a) Injury presents as muscle atrophy and limited shoulder movement.
- Lateral pectoral nerve: innervates the pectoralis major.
    (a) Injury presents as atrophy of the pectoralis major and limitation of shoulder movement.
- Intercostobrachial nerve: originates as a lateral cutaneous branch of the second intercostal nerve, supplies sensory innervation to the medial aspect of the upper arm.
    (a) Injury presents as numbness and pain of the upper inner arm.

Surgical Approaches

Lumpectomy

Lumpectomy, also called partial mastectomy or breast-conserving surgery (BCS), is a procedure in which the goal is complete excision of the breast disease with a rim of normal tissue (i.e., negative margin). Identification of the area of intended resection can be guided either by palpation or, in the case of non-palpable disease, by any number of an array of localization techniques. Regardless of the method of localization, the general steps of the operation are the same [5].

1. Identify the appropriate incision based on the location of the mass.
    (a) Incision choice is guided by cosmetic considerations (periareolar and incisions within natural skin creases are preferred) and to ensure appropriate resection.
2. Raise tissue flaps at an appropriate depth to gain access to the tumor, guided by localization technique or palpation.
3. Remove the specimen.
4. Perform intra-operative imaging to verify presence of localization marker (if relevant) and biopsy clip in the specimen.
5. Take additional shave margins and place radio-opaque clips in the cavity to guide radiation treatment/subsequent imaging.
6. If possible, approximate the space created by the removal of the tissue to optimize the cosmetic outcome.

In most institutions, intra-operative evaluation of margins is not available, and thus surgeons and patients must wait for the final pathology report to understand if sufficient margins have been obtained (see section "Margins"). For positive, or in some cases close, margins, a re-excision procedure must be undertaken. Patients must return to the operating room, the original cavity must be re-opened, and more tissue taken from the margins that were shown to be insufficient.

Following a lumpectomy with negative margins, many patients should undergo radiation to reduce the risks of local recurrence, although omission of radiation in certain populations of women with very low-risk disease is safe. "Breast-conserving therapy" (BCT) is the term used for the combination of a lumpectomy plus radiation therapy.

Wire Localization

Stiff wires are placed through the skin and into the area of concern, typically on the day of the procedure, by a radiology team, utilizing either mammography or ultrasonography. For larger lesions (e.g., >2–3 cm), multiple wires may be placed to "bracket" the area of concern. To identify the tissue to be removed, the surgeon uses mammographic images of the wires and breast to understand the relationship between portions of the wire (e.g., the barbed end and a reinforced portion), the biopsy clip, and the known disease to guide the resection. Wire localization is becoming more limited in use as the wires can become dislodged, fracture, and it can be complex to schedule both radiology and surgical teams within an appropriate time frame.

Tag Localization

A variety of different localization devices have proliferated in recent years, such as magnetic and radioactive seeds, or radiofrequency tags. These devices are placed similarly to biopsy clips with image guidance (mammography or ultrasound) by radiologists. Placement can be performed days to weeks prior to the procedure, depending on the localization device used. Intra-operatively, the surgeon utilizes a handheld probe to find the areas of highest signal to guide the borders of resection [6].

Margins

Published margin recommendations are below, although surgeons must also use discretion when reviewing pathology reports in details, to guide decisions regarding re-excision procedures.

- DCIS: ≥2 mm
- Invasive Carcinoma: no tumor on ink

Contraindications to Lumpectomy

Absolute Contraindications:
- Pregnancy
- Anticipated unacceptable cosmetic outcome to the patient

Relative Contraindications:
- Prior radiation
- Multifocal or multicentric disease precluding a good cosmetic outcome
- Large tumor-to-breast ratio
- Inability to undergo necessary radiation
- Recurrent disease after prior whole breast radiation

In recent years, contraindications to breast conservation have become increasingly challenged, expanding the safe use of breast-conserving therapy. Patients may also elect to undergo mastectomy, as opposed to BCT, if they do not wish to undergo adjuvant radiation or if desired for peace of mind. Decisions to undergo either type of cancer resection are nuanced and require an in-depth discussion among a multidisciplinary breast oncology team as well as detailed discussions about the myriad risks, benefits, and expected outcomes between patients and surgeons.

Risks of Lumpectomy

Common risks of lumpectomy include the risk of bleeding, infection, and seroma formation. Lumpectomy also bears the risk of the need for additional surgery to re-excise margins or in the case of a missed mammographic abnormality. Patients who undergo lumpectomy may also observe a change in their breast contour or sensation on the breast.

Mastectomy

Some patients require mastectomy, and others may prefer it for a variety of reasons (e.g., to decrease the potential need for radiation, risk reduction, anxiety). In all approaches to mastectomy, the central tenet is the removal of as much glandular tissue of the breast as possible, although patients should be counseled that it is impossible to remove 100% of breast tissue. Multiple approaches are available for patients undergoing a total mastectomy, including non-skin-sparing mastectomy, nipple-sparing mastectomy, and skin-sparing mastectomy. Radical mastectomy is a largely historical technique and will not be described in more detail [7].

Simple or Total Mastectomy

A total mastectomy involves the complete resection of the breast tissue to reach its anatomic borders. Following mastectomy, patients may pursue autologous or autogenous reconstruction or opt for an aesthetic flat closure.

Key Steps:

1. Make an elliptical incision over the center of the breast, including the nipple-areolar complex and skin.
   (a) Nipple-sparing mastectomy may be performed through alternative incisions including an inframammary, midlateral, peri-areolar, or combination depending on anatomy and surgeon preference.
2. Raise uniform mastectomy flaps in the "mastectomy plane," taking care not to expose the dermis, but doing as complete a resection as possible of all breast tissue as possible, radiating outwards from the incision.
3. Flaps should extend to the clavicle superiorly, lateral edge of the sternum medially, inframammary fold inferiorly, and anterior edge of the latissimus dorsi laterally.
4. Once the entire breast is separated away from the skin, remove the breast from the underlying pectoralis muscle.
   (a) The fascia of the pectoralis muscle may or may not be removed as well depending on surgeon preference.
   (b) The fascia overlying the serratus anterior is often preserved to aid with reconstructive surgery.
5. Orient the sample and ensure appropriate hemostasis prior to closure or reconstruction.
   (a) If completing a modified radical mastectomy, excision of level I and II axillary lymph nodes are also required at this time.

Skin-Sparing Mastectomy (SSM) and Nipple-Sparing Mastectomy (NSM)

For patients with suitable margins, SSM and NSM can help to facilitate improved cosmetic outcomes. Each approach preserves more breast skin than a total mastectomy as well as the infra-mammary fold [8]. The steps are like that of a total mastectomy; however, SSM includes resection of a smaller ellipse of skin while NSM preserves the nipple-areolar complex as well as the skin overlying the breast. When performing NSM, it is especially important to ensure removal of all breast tissue posterior to the nipple and to send an additional "nipple margin" pathologic specimen [9]. A positive nipple margin is usually an indication for nipple resection. Patients who have undergone either skin-sparing mastectomy or nipple-sparing mastectomy should be evaluated post-operatively for necrosis of the preserved tissue as blood flow is easily compromised by too thin flaps or hematoma/seroma formation.

Inflammatory breast cancer is a contraindication for SSM and NSM, and direct nipple involvement such as Paget's disease of the breast, is a contraindication to NSM.

Contraindications to Mastectomy

There are relatively few contraindications to mastectomy; however, patients with known metastatic disease or the inability to tolerate general anesthesia are poor candidates.

Risks of Mastectomy

Similarly to lumpectomy, mastectomy bears risks of bleeding, infection, and change in sensation. Women who undergo mastectomy may also experience flap or nipple necrosis, chronic pain, or chronic seroma formation.

Reconstruction

Post-Lumpectomy Reconstruction

Oncoplastic Reduction

Patients undergoing lumpectomy are eligible for a range of approaches considered "oncoplastic" surgery. Surgical treatments can include a contralateral reduction to maintain symmetry, bilateral lift procedures, or a range of approaches to bring superior cosmetic outcomes. Oncoplastic procedures are typically performed concurrently with lumpectomy.

Volume Replacement

Local flaps can also be used to fill in defects in certain parts of the breast. For example, a lateral intercostal artery perforator (LICAP) flap involves harvesting of skin and fat inferior to the axilla, with careful attention to preserve the lateral intercostal artery perforator. The tissue, with its intact blood supply, can be rotated into the breast to fill defects in the upper outer quadrant. Other local flaps can be used to fill defects in the inferior parts of the breast, such as thoracoepigastric flaps.

Post-Mastectomy Reconstruction

Timing

- Immediate reconstruction occurs at the same time as the mastectomy and is generally preferred. Immediate reconstruction saves the patient an additional operation and results in better condition of the skin overlying the breast. Inflammatory breast cancer is a contraindication to immediate breast reconstruction.
- Delayed reconstruction, on the other hand, occurs after healing from the mastectomy. Either implant or autologous reconstruction can be performed in an immediate or delayed fashion depending on patient factors.

Implant-Based Reconstruction

Implant-based reconstruction can provide patient satisfaction and restore body image. Implant reconstruction can be performed either in two stages, with the use of tissue expander followed by implant placement, or in one stage, termed "direct to implant." Placement of a tissue expander occurs at the time of the mastectomy followed by sequential injection of saline into the expander roughly every 2 weeks for 4–6 weeks. Following a roughly 3-month period of expansion, an implant reconstruction would subsequently be performed. Tissue expanders are used to prevent compromise of the skin after the mastectomy by reducing tension immediately postoperatively, expanders can also help to increase the size of the cavity to accommodate a larger implant. Direct to implant reconstruction, on the other hand, is performed at the time of the mastectomy and is most suitable for women undergoing NSM or SSM and who are receiving relatively light implants.

Technical considerations include location and type of implant. Implants may be placed either in front of or behind the pectoral muscle. Subpectoral implants are protective for the skin and potentially more aesthetically favorable. For pre-pectoral implants, surgeons may consider fat grafting from other areas of the body to improve appearance of the implant and to create a smooth contour. Additional considerations in implant-based reconstruction include the type of the implant: silicone looks and feels more like native breast tissue but requires more monitoring for leaks, as they may be subtle, and has greater safety concerns than saline implants.

Risks of Implant-Based Reconstruction

In addition to the complications of mastectomy, implant reconstruction bears a higher risk of infection due to the introduction of foreign materials. These infections can require the removal of the implant. Patients who receive subpectoral implants may develop altered function of the muscle, though this risk may be more theoretical than appreciated by patients.

Implant reconstruction provides less durable cosmetic result than other approaches. Roughly 1/3 of patients who receive a direct to implant reconstruction require additional procedures in the future to address cosmesis or remove the implant. In the long term, patients may develop scar tissue around the implant leading to capsular contraction and a loss of symmetry requiring additional intervention. This risk of this complication is higher in women who receive radiation. Additionally, patients who receive implant reconstruction require monitoring for implant leakage which occurs for patients with silicone implants at a rate of 1% per year.

Systemic risks associated with implant-based reconstruction include breast implant associated anaplastic large cell lymphoma (ALCL) and breast implant illness (BII). ALCL is associated with the use of textured implants, which have been removed from the market by the FDA; however, women with a history of reconstruction should be assessed. BII is a constellation of symptoms possible among women who have implants, either for reconstruction or augmentation, including fatigue, brain fog, myalgias, or rashes. BII is rare and more common among patients who have had implants for augmentation and appears to resolve with removal of the implants.

Autologous Tissue Reconstruction

The most common source of tissue for autologous reconstruction is the lower abdomen, either via a deep inferior epigastric perforator flap (DIEP) or transverse rectus abdominus myocutaneous flaps (TRAM) flap. The key difference is the degree of involvement of the rectus abdominus, for which the DIEP approach causes less tissue trauma. In either approach, a section of fat and blood vessels is removed from the lower abdomen (similar to a tummy-tuck procedure) and transferred to the chest where the mastectomy has been performed. The reconstructive surgeon then shapes the transferred tissue into a breast. Autologous reconstruction generally has more durable cosmetic outcomes than implant-based reconstruction.

Risks of Autologous Reconstruction

Autologous reconstruction is a longer operation than implant-based reconstruction, typically lasting 6–8 h for a single breast. In addition to complications of mastectomy and more prolonged anesthetic time, patients who choose autologous reconstruction may experience changes in sensation and function in the abdominal area as well as the breast. These patients will require a longer period of recovery due to the additional area of intervention. Women with autologous reconstruction may also require additional procedures in the future, including liposuction of the abdominal tissues which may increase in size disproportionately to the breast tissue if patients gain weight.

Surgical Management of the Axilla

Exploration of the lymphatic drainage of the breast may be indicated for staging and prognostic purposes. It is important to note that axillary management does not always have a therapeutic role. Axillary lymph node dissection (ALND) has largely been replaced by sentinel lymph node biopsy (SLNBx) in the treatment of early-stage breast cancer but is still relevant for women with locally advanced disease. Inflammatory breast cancer is a contraindication to SLNBx as it requires an ALND. Axillary surgery can be associated with significant morbidity related to lymphedema and nerve injury, driving efforts to limit overtreatment.

Sentinel Lymph Node Biopsy (SLNB)

SLNB allows surgeons to minimize the morbidity of axillary dissection while still gaining important prognostic and therapeutic information. SLNB is indicated in most patients with invasive breast cancer and a clinically negative axilla or for patients undergoing a mastectomy for high-risk lesions, including DCIS, as the drainage system will be disrupted by the procedure and subsequent SLNB will not be feasible. SLNB requires the use of a tracer, typically a radio-tracer (technetium-99m), blue dye (isosulfan blue or methylene blue), or, a combined technique. Of note, isosulfan blue dye has been associated with anaphylaxis (0.5% risk), can result in permanent discoloration of the skin if injected into the dermis, and is contraindicated in pregnancy.

Key Steps:
1. Inject radiotracer into the site of the tumor, in the subareolar plexus, or in the dermis at the nipple; blue dye can also be injected in the subareolar plexus.
2. Either a separate curvilinear incision at the bottom of the hair-bearing axillary skin can be made or the procedure may be carried out through the lumpectomy/mastectomy incision.

3. Utilize a gamma probe to determine the location of the probable sentinel node.
4. Dissect down to the clavipectoral fascia.
5. Identify the hottest node (based on gamma probe count) and excise it.
6. Remove any additional nodes with greater than 10% the count of the hottest node, nodes which are blue, or any palpable nodes.
7. Drains do not need to be routinely left.
8. Close the incision.

Risks of SLNB

Risks of SLNB include the risk of bleeding, infection, change in sensation, nerve or vascular injury, and seroma formation. Additional risks include a false negative result, which use of dual mapping techniques aims to reduce. Finally, 3–7% of patients who undergo SLNB will develop lymphedema.

Axillary Lymph Node Dissection (ALND)

Complete axillary lymph node dissection is indicated for patients with T4 or inflammatory breast cancer, occult cancer with known axillary metastasis, failed mapping, axillary recurrence, or patients with positive nodes after neoadjuvant chemotherapy. Complete axillary dissection is also usually necessary in patients with clinical node positivity [10], although there are some cases in which a SLNB may be appropriate as a first step. Axillary lymph node dissections for breast cancer include only level I and level II nodes, unless level III nodes are grossly involved.

Key Steps:
1. Make a curvilinear incision at the inferior edge of the hair bearing skin of the axilla extending within the curve of the axilla from the pectoralis major to the medial border of the latissimus dorsi.
2. Utilizing electrocautery, dissect through the subcutaneous tissue and raise skin flaps with the inferior flap raised to approximately the level of the fourth or fifth rib.
3. Incise the pectoralis fascia to raise the pectoralis major and visualize levels II and III.
4. Identify major landmarks: the axillary vein superiorly, the medial pectoral bundle, the long thoracic nerve along the chest wall, and the thoracodorsal bundle. The thoracoepigastric vein, which is usually anterior to the thoracodorsal vein, can be ligated as part of this procedure. If possible, branches of the intercostobrachial nerve should be preserved, although they can be ligated for the purposes of completing the procedure.

5. Remove the nodal tissue, irrigate the wound, and ensure hemostasis.
6. A drain is typically left in place to decrease post-operative seromas.
7. Close the incision.

Risks of ALND

Risks of ALND are the same as those for SLNB; however, the risk of lymphedema is significantly increased to 15–25% of patients.

Male Breast Cancer

Men make up <1% of breast cancer diagnoses and are usually diagnosed via palpable findings. Although most males in the past have undergone mastectomy due to the subareolar nature of the majority of male breast cancers and the relative paucity of breast tissue, men can still choose between breast conservation and mastectomy. The technical approaches are the same as for women.

Conclusions

The surgical management of non-metastatic breast cancer continues to evolve quickly as indications for breast conservation (with or without accompanying oncoplastic techniques) and SLNB (instead of ALND), and even omission of axillary surgery altogether, grow. Careful attention must be paid to clinical trial data that inform the nuances of treatment decision-making to ensure that patients are receiving appropriate counseling to help them make informed decisions about their care.

References

1. SEER. Cancer of the breast (female) – cancer stat facts. 2025. Available at: https://seer.cancer.gov/statfacts/html/breast.html. Accessed 3 Jan 2025.
2. Czajka ML, Pfeifer C. Breast cancer surgery. In: StatPearls [Internet]. StatPearls Publishing; 2023. Available at: https://www.ncbi.nlm.nih.gov/sites/books/NBK553076/. Accessed 7 Jan 2025.
3. Pandya S, Moore RG. Breast development and anatomy. Clin Obstet Gynecol. 2011;54(1):91–5. Available at: https://doi.org/10.1097/GRF.0b013e318207ffe9.
4. Rivard AB, Galarza-Paez L, Peterson DC. Anatomy, thorax, breast. In: StatPearls. Treasure Island: StatPearls Publishing; 2024. Available at: http://www.ncbi.nlm.nih.gov/books/NBK519575/. Accessed 19 Dec 2024.

5. Rahman GA. Breast conserving therapy: a surgical technique where little can mean more. J Surg Tech Case Rep. 2011;3(1):1–4. Available at: https://doi.org/10.4103/2006-8808.78459.
6. Kapoor MM, Patel MM, Scoggins ME. The wire and beyond: recent advances in breast imaging preoperative needle localization. Radiographics. 2019;39(7):1886–906. Available at: https://doi.org/10.1148/rg.2019190041.
7. Freeman MD, Gopman JM, Salzberg CA. The evolution of mastectomy surgical technique: from mutilation to medicine. Gland Surg. 2018;7(3):308–15. Available at: https://doi.org/10.21037/gs.2017.09.07.
8. Seth I, et al. Defining skin-sparing mastectomy surgical techniques: a narrative review. Ann Breast Surg. 2024;8:20. Available at: https://doi.org/10.21037/abs-23-19.
9. The American Society of Breast Surgeons. Resource guide for mastectomy. 2014. Available at: https://www.breastsurgeons.org/docs/statements/asbrs-rg-mastectomy.pdf. Accessed 19 Dec 2024.
10. Themes UFO. Axillary lymph node dissection. Oncohema Key. 14 Jan 2019. Available at: https://oncohemakey.com/axillary-lymph-node-dissection/. Accessed 7 Jan 2025.

Chapter 5
Breast Cancer-Related Lymphedema

Erin M. Taylor

Lymphedema

Lymphedema is a chronic, progressive disease of lymphatic system insufficiency that leads to accumulation of lymphatic fluid in the interstitial space of the surrounding tissues.

- Over time, this process can result in significant swelling and functional impairment of the affected limb.
- Lymphedema can lead to significant physical, psychological, and financial burden to patients resulting in reduced quality of life [1].

Primary lymphedema is lymphedema caused by impairment of the lymphatic system at birth.

Secondary lymphedema is caused by subsequent damage of the lymphatic system after birth.

- Secondary lymphedema can be caused by infection (most commonly filariasis worldwide), surgery, trauma, obesity, radiation therapy, and medical therapies.
- In developed countries, secondary lymphedema is most commonly caused by *oncologic treatment*.
- In the United States, upper extremity lymphedema most commonly develops as a complication of breast cancer treatment, known as *breast cancer-related lymphedema (BCRL)*.

E. M. Taylor (✉)
Brigham and Women's Hospital, Harvard Medical School, Boston, MA, USA
e-mail: etaylor@bwh.harvard.edu

Breast Cancer-Related Lymphedema

The lifetime risk of breast cancer for women in the United States is approximately 1 in 8 [2]. Of those treated for breast cancer, an estimated 1 in 5 will develop breast cancer-related lymphedema [3].

Treatment of breast cancer often involves lumpectomy and radiation therapy (breast-conserving therapy) versus mastectomy. At the time of lumpectomy or mastectomy, lymph nodes are removed with either *sentinel lymph node biopsy* (SLNB) or *axillary lymph node dissection* (ALND), which involves a greater number of lymph nodes removed. Additional treatments include post-mastectomy radiation therapy (PMRT), hormone-based therapy, immunotherapy, and chemotherapy, which can be neoadjuvant or adjuvant. Type of breast cancer treatment significantly impacts the risk of developing breast cancer-related lymphedema.

Risk of Breast Cancer-Related Lymphedema

Oncologic Treatment Impact on BCRL

The risk of breast cancer-related lymphedema (BCRL) varies based on the required oncologic treatments.

- The rate of lymphedema increases with *number of lymph nodes removed, radiation therapy, and chemotherapy*.
- While modern oncologic treatments are highly effective at treating breast cancer, numerous studies have associated *axillary lymph node dissection (ALND)*, *post-mastectomy radiation therapy (PMRT)*, and *taxane-based chemotherapy* as major risk factors for developing lymphedema [4, 5].
- Patients undergoing mastectomy, ALND, and post-mastectomy radiation therapy have a *30–40% risk of lymphedema*.
- Type of breast cancer also impacts rate of lymphedema development.
- Inflammatory breast cancer has the highest rate of lymphedema at 50.6% [6].

Sentinel Lymph Node Biopsy (SLNB) Axilla—5–7%
Axillary Lymph Node Dissection (ALND)—25–35%
ALND + Radiation Therapy—25–40%
Adjuvant chemotherapy + ALND—HR 2.7
Taxol chemotherapy + ALND—HR 3.8
Inflammatory Breast Cancer—50.6%

Patient Characteristics Impact on BCRL

Additional risk factors have been associated with patient characteristics.

Obesity

- Obesity has independently been associated with higher rates of lymphedema in patients without cancer diagnoses [7, 8].
- Studies on BCRL have found higher body mass index (BMI) associated with higher rates of lymphedema [9, 10].

Race/Ethnicity

- Smaller studies on BCRL suggest that race impacts the risk of lymphedema development.
- Patients of Black and Hispanic backgrounds have been associated with increased rates of lymphedema after breast cancer treatment [11–13].

Prevention of Breast Cancer-Related Lymphedema

Due to the recalcitrant nature of lymphedema to treatment, prevention of breast cancer-related lymphedema is the goal.

Nonsurgical Prevention

- The most widely used method for prevention and treatment of breast cancer-related lymphedema is *complex decongestive therapy (CDT)*.
- CDT uses a combination of manual lymphatic drainage, compression sleeves, exercise, pneumatic compression, and skin care to improve lymphatic drainage of the affected extremity.

Surgical Prevention

- *Immediate lymphatic reconstruction (ILR)* with lymphovenous bypass at the time of axillary lymph node dissection offers a preventative option for patients at high risk for breast cancer-related lymphedema.

- *Lymphovenous bypass (LVB)* involves performing a series of lymphovenous anastomoses on freshly transected lymphatic vessels to redirect the flow of lymphatic fluid back into the venous system.
- A meta-analysis by *Chang* et al. [14] found prophylactic lymphovenous bypass reduces the incidence of lymphedema.
- Corridi et al. [15] reported preliminary results of a randomized control trial that ILR at the time of ALND in high-risk patients reduced the rate of BCRL to from 30% to 9%.

Treatment of Breast Cancer-Related Lymphedema

Conservative treatment with complete decongestive therapy (CDT) is performed prior to proceeding with lymphatic surgery. If conservative therapy is not sufficient to treat lymphedema alone, surgical treatment can be performed after CDT optimization of lymphedema symptoms.

Depending on the stage of lymphedema, surgical options for lymphedema treatment include physiologic or debulking procedures.

Early-stage lymphedema is characterized by pitting edema, dermal backflow, and extracellular fluid. Physiologic procedures are performed with goal to reverse effects of early-stage lymphedema with improved lymphatic flow.

Late-stage lymphedema is characterized by fibrofatty deposition. Debulking procedures such as liposuction target areas of fibrofatty deposition for surgical removal of fibrofatty tissue.

Nonsurgical Treatment

- *Complex decongestive therapy (CDT)* uses a combination of manual lymphatic drainage, compression sleeves, exercise, and skin care to improve lymphatic drainage of the affected extremity.
- While CDT can reduce symptoms in many patients, it requires long-term adherence that patients may find burdensome and is most effective during early-stage disease [16].
- Accordingly, a recent systematic review of quality-of-life outcomes by *Fish* et al. found that CDT was associated with mixed patient-reported outcomes [17].

Surgical Treatment

- Lymphatic surgery offers an option to patients for whom conservative therapy is ineffective.

- For early-stage lymphedema, physiologic procedures can be performed with goal to improve lymphatic outflow from the effected extremity and decrease limb volume.
- For late-stage lymphedema, debulking procedures can be performed to remove fibrofatty tissue and reduce limb volume.

Physiologic Procedures

- Options of lymphatic surgery for the treatment of early-stage lymphedema include *lymphovenous bypass (LVB)* and *vascularized lymph node transplant (VLNT)*.
- A meta-analysis found LVB and VLNT to be effective treatment options for patients with early-stage lymphedema [14].

Lymphovenous Bypass

- *Lymphovenous bypass (LVB)* involves performing a series of anastomoses between lymph channels to nearby veins.
- Lymphovenous bypasses redirect the flow of lymphatic fluid back into the venous system distal to an area of dermal backflow.

Vascularized Lymph Node Transplant

- *Vascularized lymph node transplant (VLNT)* transfers lymph nodes from the lymph node donor site to the axilla or affected extremity as a free flap.
- Donor sites include the greater omentum, superficial groin, supraclavicular lymph nodes, and submental lymph nodes.
- VLNT has been found to reduce limb volume and improve patient reported outcomes by 2-years postoperative [18].

Debulking Procedures

For patients with advanced stage lymphedema, debulking procedures can be performed to reduce limb volume.

Liposuction

- Liposuction with combination of compression therapy effectively reduces limb volume.
- Typically preferred treatment for late-stage lymphedema over direct excision.

Direct Excision

- Direct excision of subcutaneous limb tissue followed by tissue advancement or skin grafting can effectively reduce limb volume.
- Now rarely performed due to morbidity.

References

1. Fu MR, Kang Y. Psychosocial impact of living with cancer-related lymphedema. Semin Oncol Nurs. 2013;29(1):50–60. https://doi.org/10.1016/j.soncn.2012.11.007.
2. DeSantis CE, Ma J, Gaudet MM, Newman LA, Miller KD, Goding Sauer A, Jemal A, Siegel RL. Breast cancer statistics, 2019. CA Cancer J Clin. 2019;69(6):438–51. https://doi.org/10.3322/caac.21583.
3. Ridner SH. Pathophysiology of lymphedema. Semin Oncol Nurs. 2013;29(1):4–11. https://doi.org/10.1016/j.soncn.2012.11.002.
4. Aoishi Y, Oura S, Nishiguchi H, Hirai Y, Miyasaka M, Kawaji M, Shima A, Nishimura Y. Risk factors for breast cancer-related lymphedema: correlation with docetaxel administration. Breast Cancer. 2020;27(5):929–37. https://doi.org/10.1007/s12282-020-01088-x.
5. Koelmeyer LA, Gaitatzis K, Dietrich MS, Shah CS, Boyages J, McLaughlin SA, Taback B, Stolldorf DP, Elder E, Hughes TM, French JR, Ngui N, Hsu JM, Moore A, Ridner SH. Risk factors for breast cancer-related lymphedema in patients undergoing 3 years of prospective surveillance with intervention. Cancer. 2022;128:3408–15. https://doi.org/10.1002/cncr.34377.
6. Farley CR, Irwin S, Adesoye T, et al. Lymphedema in inflammatory breast cancer patients following trimodal treatment. Ann Surg Oncol. 2022;29(10):6370–8. https://doi.org/10.1245/s10434-022-12142-7.
7. Mehrara B, Greene A. Lymphedema and obesity: is there a link? Plast Reconstr Surg. 2014;134(1):154e–60e.
8. Sudduth C, Greene A. Lymphedema and obesity. Cold Spring Harb Perspect Med. 2023;12(5):2157–1422.
9. Boyages J, Cave A, Naidoo D, Ee C. Weight gain and lymphedema after breast cancer treatment: avoiding the catch-22? Lymphat Res Biol. 2022;20(4):409–16.
10. Tsai R, Dennis L, Lynch C, Snetselaar L, Zamba G, Scott-Conner C. Lymphedema following breast cancer: the importance of surgical methods and obesity. Front Womens Health. 2018;3(2):1–17.
11. Kwan M, Yao S, Lee V, Roh J, Zhu Q, Ergas I, Liu Q, Zhang Y, Kutner S, Quesenberry C, Ambrozone C, Kushi L. Race/ethnicity, genetic ancestry, and breast cancer-related lymphedema in the pathways study. Breast Cancer Res Treat. 2016;159:119–29.
12. Montagna G, Zhang J, Sevilimedu V, Charyn J, Abbate K, Gomez E, Mehrara B, Morrow M, Barrio A. Risk factors and racial and ethnic disparities in patients with breast cancer-related lymphedema. JAMA Oncol. 2022;8(8):1195–200.

13. Yumeng R, Kebede M, Ogunleye A, Emerson M, Evenson K, Carey L, Hayes S, Troester M. Burden of lymphedema in long-term breast cancer survivors by race and age. Cancer. 2022;128:4119–28.
14. Chang DW, Dayan J, Greene AK, MacDonald JK, Masia J, Mehrara B, Neligan PC, Nguyen D. Surgical treatment of lymphedema: a systematic review and meta-analysis of controlled trials. Results of a consensus conference. Plast Reconstr Surg. 2021;147(4):975–93. https://doi.org/10.1097/PRS.0000000000007783.
15. Coriddi M, Dayan J, Bloomfield E, et al. Efficacy of immediate lymphatic reconstruction to decrease incidence of breast cancer-related lymphedema: preliminary results of randomized controlled trial. Ann Surg. 2023;278(4):630–7. https://doi.org/10.1097/SLA.0000000000005952.
16. Smile TD, Tendulkar R, Schwarz G, Arthur D, Grobmyer S, Valente S, Vicini F, Shah C. A review of treatment for breast cancer-related lymphedema: paradigms for clinical practice. Am J Clin Oncol. 2018;41(2):178–90. https://doi.org/10.1097/COC.0000000000000355.
17. Fish ML, Grover R, Schwarz GS. Quality-of-life outcomes in surgical vs nonsurgical treatment of breast cancer-related lymphedema: a systematic review. JAMA Surg. 2020;155(6):513–9. https://doi.org/10.1001/jamasurg.2020.0230.
18. Brown S, Mehrara BJ, Coriddi M, McGrath L, Cavalli M, Dayan JH. A prospective study on the safety and efficacy of vascularized lymph node transplant. Ann Surg. 2022;276(4):635–53. https://doi.org/10.1097/SLA.0000000000005591.

Index

A
Anaplastic large cell lymphoma (ALCL), 50
Architectural distortion, 31
Asymmetries, 31
Atypical ductal hyperplasia (ADH)
   biopsy diagnosis of, 9
   and future breast cancer risk
      implications, 9
   incidence and epidemiology, 7, 8
   and low-grade DCIS, 8
Atypical papilloma, 13
   biopsy diagnosis of, 14
   and future breast cancer risk
      implications, 14
   incidence and epidemiology, 13
Autologous tissue reconstruction, 50
   risks of, 51
Axilla
   anatomic boundaries of, 43
   nerves and potential effects of nerve injury
      in, 43, 44
   surgical management of, 51
      axillary lymph node dissection, 52, 53
      sentinel lymph node biopsy, 51, 52
Axillary lymph node dissection (ALND),
      51–53, 56
   risks of, 53
Axillary lymph nodes, 43

B
Benign breast cysts
   complicated cysts, 2
   simple cysts, 1
Benign phyllodes, 3

Benign/physiologic nipple discharge, 5
Borderline phyllodes, 3, 4
Breast
   anatomic boundaries of, 42
   anatomy of, 42–44
Breast cancer, 41
   autologous tissue reconstruction, 50
      risks of, 51
   axilla
      anatomic boundaries of, 43
      axillary lymph node dissection, 53
      axillary lymph nodes, 43
      nerves and potential effects of nerve
         injury in, 43, 44
      surgical management of, 51–53
   blood supply, 42, 43
   implant-based reconstruction, 49, 50
      risks of, 50
   male breast cancer, 53
   post-lumpectomy reconstruction
      oncoplastic reduction, 48, 49
      volume replacement, 49
   post-mastectomy reconstruction, 49
   surgical approaches
      lumpectomy, 44–46
      mastectomy, 47, 48
Breast cancer risk reduction
   chemotherapeutic agents for, 10
Breast cancer-related lymphedema
      (BCRL), 55, 56
   Debulking procedures, 59
   direct excision, 60
   liposuction, 60
   lymphedema, 55
   lymphovenous bypass, 59

Breast cancer-related lymphedema (BCRL) (cont.)
  non-surgical prevention, 57
  non-surgical treatment, 58
  physiologic procedures, 59
  prevention of, 57
  risk of
    obesity, 57
    oncologic treatment impact on, 56
    patient characteristics impact on, 57
    race/ethnicity, 57
  surgical prevention, 57, 58
  surgical treatment, 58
  treatment of, 58
  vascularized lymph node transplant, 59
Breast imaging, screening in
  biopsy modalities, 38
  breast imaging-reporting and data system, 36, 37
  breast MRI, 24, 25
  contrast-enhanced mammography, 24
  diagnostic contrast enhanced mammography, 36
  diagnostic mammography
    architectural distortion, 28, 31
    asymmetries, 31
    calcifications, types of, 29, 30
    indications, 26
    mass, 28
    supplemental views, 31–32
  diagnostic ultrasound, 32, 33
    calcifications, 34
    indications, 34, 35
  mammography, 17
    average risk patients, 23
    breast composition, 21
    breast imaging reporting and data system, 22
    clockface notation, 20
    digital breast tomosynthesis, 19
    high-risk patients, 23
    imaging views, 17
    localization, 19
    mean glandular dose, 20
    quadrants, 20
    recommendations for screening, 22, 23
    standard views, 18
  molecular breast imaging /breast-specific gamma imaging, 25
Breast Imaging-Reporting and Data System (BI-RADS®), 36, 37

Breast implant illness (BII), s, 50
Breast MRI, 24, 25
Breast-specific gamma imaging (BSGI), 25

C
Calcifications, 29–31
Complex decongestive therapy (CDT), 57, 58
Complicated cysts, 2
Contrast-enhanced mammography (CEM), 24

D
Debulking procedures, 59
Diagnostic contrast enhanced mammography, 36
Diagnostic mammography
  architectural distortion, 28, 31
  asymmetries, 31
  calcifications, types of, 29, 30
  indications, 26
  mass, 28
  supplemental views, 31–32
Diagnostic ultrasound, 32, 33
  calcifications, 34
  indications, 34, 35
Digital breast tomosynthesis (DBT), 19
Direct excision, 60
Distribution patterns, 30–31
Duct ectasia, 5
Ductal carcinoma in situ (DCIS), 5

E
Early-stage lymphedema, 58

F
Fibroadenomas, 2, 3
Fibroepithelial neoplasms
  benign phyllodes, 3
  borderline phyllodes, 3, 4
  fibroadenomas, 2, 3
  malignant phyllodes, 4
  phyllodes tumors, 3
Florid LCIS, 12

I
Immediate lymphatic reconstruction (ILR), 57
Implant-based reconstruction, 49, 50

Index

risks of, 50
Infected montgomery's gland, 4

L
Liposuction, 60
Lobular neoplasia (LN)
  atypical Papilloma
    biopsy diagnosis of, 14
    and future breast cancer risk
      implications, 14
    incidence and epidemiology, 13
  biopsy diagnosis of, 11
  florid and pleomorphic LCIS
    biopsy diagnosis of, 12
    and future breast cancer risk
      implications, 13
    incidence and epidemiology, 12
  and future breast cancer risk
    implications, 11
  incidence and epidemiology, 10
Lower inner quadrant (LIQ), 20
Lower outer quadrant (LOQ), 20
Lumpectomy, 44, 45
  contraindications to, 46
  margin, 46
  risks of, 46
  tag localization, 45
  wire localization, 45
Lymphedema, 55
Lymphovenous bypass (LVB), 58, 59

M
Male breast cancer, 53
Malignant phyllodes, 4
Mammography
  breast imaging, screening, 17
    average risk patients, 23
    breast composition, 21
    Breast Imaging Reporting and Data
      System, 22
    clockface notation, 20
    digital breast tomosynthesis, 19
    high-risk patients, 23
    imaging views, 17
    localization, 19
    mean glandular dose, 20
    quadrants, 20
    recommendations for
      screening, 22, 23
    standard views, 18
Mastectomy, 47
  contraindications, 48
  risks of, 48
  simple/total mastectomy, 47
  skin sparing mastectomy and nipple
    sparing mastectomy, 48
Mean glandular dose (MGD), 20
Molecular breast imaging, 25

N
Nipple discharge, 5
  benign/physiologic, 5
  pathologic, 5
Non-spontaneous nipple discharge, 5

O
Obesity, 57
Oncoplastic reduction, 48–49

P
Papillomas, 5
Pathologic nipple discharge, 5
Periareolar abscess
  infected montgomery's
    gland, 4
  periductal fistula, 4, 5
Periductal fistula, 4, 5
Phyllodes tumors, 3
Pleomorphic LCIS, 12
Post-lumpectomy reconstruction
  oncoplastic reduction, 48, 49
  volume replacement, 49
Post-mastectomy reconstruction, 49
Primary lymphedema, 55
Prolactin, 5

Q
Quadrants, 20

R
Race/ethnicity, 57

S
Secondary lymphedema, 55

Sentinel lymph node biopsy (SLNB),
    51–52, 56
  risks of, 52
Simple cysts, 1
Spontaneous nipple discharge, 5

T
3D mammography, 19

U
Upper inner quadrant (UIQ), 20
Upper outer quadrant (UOQ), 20

V
Vascularized lymph node transplant
    (VLNT), 59

If you have any concerns about our products,
you can contact us on
ProductSafety@springernature.com

In case Publisher is established outside the EU,
the EU authorized representative is:
**Springer Nature Customer Service Center GmbH
Europaplatz 3, 69115 Heidelberg, Germany**

Printed by Libri Plureos GmbH
in Hamburg, Germany